FEMA 427 / *December 2003*

RISK MANAGEMENT SERIES

I0118905

Primer *for* Design of Commercial Buildings to Mitigate Terrorist Attacks

PROVIDING PROTECTION TO PEOPLE AND BUILDINGS

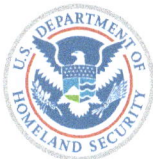

FEMA

Federal Emergency Management Agency
www.fema.gov

Published by Books Express Publishing, 2012
ISBN 978-1-78266-140-5

Books Express publications are available from all good retail and online booksellers. For
publishing proposals and direct ordering please contact us at: info@books-express.com

FOREWORD AND ACKNOWLEDGMENTS

This *Primer for Design of Commercial Buildings to Mitigate Terrorist Attacks – Protecting Office, Retail, Multi-Family Residential, and Light-Industrial Facilities,* provides guidance to building designers, owners and state and local governments to mitigate the effects of hazards resulting from terrorist attacks on new buildings. While the guidance provided focuses principally on explosive attacks and design strategies to mitigate the effects of explosions, the document also addresses design strategies to mitigate the effects of chemical, biological and radiological attacks. In addition to applicability to the design of new commercial office, retail, multi-family residential, and light-industrial buildings, many of the concepts presented are also applicable to other building types and/or existing buildings.

ACKNOWLEDGEMENTS

Principal Author:

    Applied Technology Council (ATC)

    Eve Hinman, Hinman Consulting Engineers

Contributors:

    Christopher Rojahn, Applied Technology Council

    Robert Smilowitz, Weidlinger Associates

    Kenneth Mead, Centers for Disease Control and Prevention/
        National Institute for Occupational Safety and Health

    Dominic Campi, Rutherford & Chekene

    Randy J. Meyers, Flack + Kutz Inc.

    Nancy Sauer, Rdd Consultants

    Peter Mork, Applied Technology Council

Project Advisory Panel:

    Christopher Arnold, Building Systems Development, Inc.

    Wade Belcher, General Services Administration

    Curt Betts, U. S. Army Corps of Engineers

    Jim Caulder, U. S. Air Force – Civil Engineer Support Agency

    Michael Chipley, UTD, Inc.

    Marcelle Habibion, Department of Veterans Affairs

    Joseph Hartman, U. S. Army Corps of Engineers

    David Hattis, Building Technology, Inc.

    Rick Jones, Naval Facilities Engineering Service Center

    Kurt Knight, Department of Veterans Affairs

    Frederick Krimgold, Virginia Tech

    Eric Letvin, URS Corporation

    John Lynch, Naval Facilities Command (NAVFAC) Criteria Office

    Wesley Lyon, UTD, Inc.

    Terry Pruitt, Department of Homeland Security

    Lloyd Siegel, Department of Veterans Affairs

    William Whiddon, Building Technology, Inc.

Project Officer:

> Milagros Kennett, FEMA
> > Building Sciences Technology Branch
> > Mitigation Division

This manual will be revised periodically, and comments and feedback to improve future editions are welcome. Please send comments and feedback by e-mail to riskmanagementseriespubs@dhs.gov

TABLE OF CONTENTS

FOREWORD AND ACKNOWLEDGMENTS iii

LIST OF FIGURES vii

LIST OF TABLES ix

FIGURE CREDITS xi

1   INTRODUCTION 1-1
1.1 Purpose and Overview 1-1
1.2 Contents and Organization of the Report 1-3
1.3 Further Reading 1-4

2   TERRORIST THREATS 2-1
2.1 Overview of Possible Threats 2-1
2.2 Explosive Attacks 2-1
2.3 Further Reading 2-4

3   WEAPONS EFFECTS 3-1
3.1 Description of Explosion Forces 3-1
3.2 Further Reading 3-3

4   BUILDING DAMAGE 4-1
4.1 Predicting Damage Levels 4-1
4.2 Damage Mechanisms 4-1
4.3 Correlation Between Damage and Injuries 4-5
4.4 Further Reading 4-8

5   DESIGN APPROACH 5-1
5.1 Goals of the Design Approach 5-1
5.2 Security Principles 5-2
5.3 Further Reading 5-5

6   DESIGN GUIDANCE 6-1
6.1 Site Location and Layout 6-1
6.2 Architectural 6-8
6.3 Structural 6-13
6.4 Building Envelope 6-26
6.5 Mechanical and Electrical Systems 6-35
6.6 Chemical, Biological, and Radiological Protection 6-41

7   OCCUPANCY TYPES 7-1
7.1 Overview 7-1
7.2 Multi-Family Residential Occupancy 7-1
7.3 Commercial Retail Space Occupancy 7-2
7.4 Light Industrial Buildings 7-3
7.5 Further Reading 7-5

8   COST CONSIDERATIONS 8-1
8.1 Initial Costs 8-1
8.2 Life-Cycle Costs 8-2
8.3 Setting Priorities 8-3
8.4 Further Reading 8-4

LIST OF FIGURES

2-1   Schematic of vehicle weapon threat parameters and definitions 2-2

3-1   Air-blast pressure time history 3-2

3-2   Plots showing pressure decay with distance 3-2

4-1   Schematic showing sequence of building damage due to a vehicle weapon 4-3

4-2   Schematics showing sequence of building damage due to a package weapon 4-4

4-3   Exterior view of Alfred P. Murrah Federal Building collapse . 4-5

4-4   Exterior view of Khobar Towers exterior wall failure 4-6

4-5   Photograph showing non-structural damage in building impacted by blast 4-7

5-1   Components of security 5-2

5-2   Schematic showing lines of defense against blast 5-4

6-1   Schematic of typical anti-ram bollard 6-4

6-2   Schematic of typical anti-ram knee wall 6-5

6-3   Schematics showing the effect of building shape on air-blast impacts 6-9

6-4   Schematics showing an example approach for improving the layout of adjacent unsecured and secured areas 6-10

6-5   Direct design process flow chart 6-17

6-6   Single-degree-of-feedom model for explosive loads. Note variation of force and displacement with time 6-18

6-7   Safe laminated-glass systems and failure modes 6-29

6-8   Plan view of test cubicle showing glass performance conditions as a function of distance from test window 6-31

6-9   Schematic showing recommended location for elevated air-intakes on exterior of building 6-44

8-1   Plots showing relationship between cost of upgrading various building components, standoff distance, and risk 8-2

LIST OF TABLES

4-1 Damage and Injuries due to Explosion Effects..................... 4-8
6-1 Performance Conditions for Windows 6-30

FIGURE CREDITS

3-1 Based on Figure 3.2, *Fundamentals of Protective Design for Conventional Weapons,* Technical Manual TM5-855-1, Headquarters, Department of the Army, Washington, D.C., 3 November 1, 1986.

4-3 Photograph courtesy of Exponent Failure Analysis Associates

4-4 Photograph courtesy of the U.S. Air Force

4-5 Photograph courtesy of U.S. Department of State

6-1 Based on Figure 3-6, *Security Engineering - Concept Design,* Army TM5-853-2, Air Force AFMAN 32-1071, Vol. 2, Department of the Army, and the Air Force, May 1994.

6-2 Based on Figure 14.9.6.1.3, *Architectural & Engineering Design Guidelines for U.S. Diplomatic Mission Buildings,* Office of Building Operations, U.S. Department of State, Washington D.C., June 1997.

6-7 From Figure 4-1, *ISC Security Design Criteria for New Federal Office Buildings and Major Modernization Projects,* The Interagency Security Committee, Washington, D.C., May 28, 2001.

6-9 *Guidance for Protecting Building Environments from Airborne Chemical, Biological, or Radiological Attacks,* Department of Health and Human Services, Centers for Disease Control and Prevention, National Institute for Occupational Safety and Health, May, 2002.

8-1 Courtesy of Joseph Smith of Applied Research Associates, Inc.

1.1   PURPOSE AND OVERVIEW

The purpose of this primer is to introduce concepts that can help building designers, owners, and state and local governments mitigate the threat of hazards resulting from terrorist attacks on new buildings. This primer specifically addresses four high-population, private-sector building types: commercial office, retail, multi-family residential, and light industrial. However, many of the concepts presented here are applicable to other building types and/or existing buildings. The focus is on explosive attack, but the text also addresses design strategies to mitigate the effects of chemical, biological, and radiological attacks.

Designing security into a building requires a complex series of trade-offs. Security concerns need to be balanced with many other design constraints such as accessibility, initial and life-cycle costs, natural hazard mitigation, fire protection, energy efficiency, and aesthetics. Because the probability of attack is very small, security measures should not interfere with daily operations of the building. On the other hand, because the effects of attack can be catastrophic, it is prudent to incorporate measures that may save lives and minimize business interruption in the unlikely event of an attack. The measures should be as unobtrusive as possible to provide an inviting, efficient environment that does not attract undue attention of potential attackers. Security design needs to be part of an overall multi-hazard approach to ensure that it does not worsen the behavior of the building in the event of a fire, earthquake, or hurricane, which are far more prevalent hazards than are terrorist attacks.

Because of the severity of the types of hazards discussed, the goals of security-oriented design are by necessity modest. With regard to explosive attacks, the focus is on a damage-limiting or damage-mitigating approach rather than a blast-resistant approach. The goal is to incorporate some reasonable measures that will enhance the life safety of the persons within the building and facilitate rescue efforts in the unlikely event of attack.

It is clear that owners are becoming interested in considering man-made hazards for a variety of reasons including the desire to:

- attract more tenants or a particular type of tenant,
- lower insurance premiums or obtain high-risk insurance,

- reduce life-cycle costs for operational security measures, and
- limit losses and business interruption.

Protection against terrorist attack is not an all-or-nothing proposition. Incremental measures taken early in design may be more fully developed at a later date. With a little forethought regarding, for instance, the space requirements needed to accommodate additional measures, the protection level can be enhanced as the need arises or the budget permits after construction is complete.

This primer strives to provide a holistic multi-disciplinary approach to security design by considering the various building systems including site, architecture, structure, mechanical and electrical systems and providing general recommendations for the design professional with little or no background in this area.

This is one of a series of five FEMA primers that address security issues in high-population, private-sector buildings. It is the intent of FEMA that these reports will assist designers, owners, and local/state government officials in gaining a solid understanding of man-made hazards. These reports will also discuss current state-of-the-art methods to enhance protection of the building by incorporating low-cost measures into new buildings at the earliest stages of site selection and design.

Best practices recommended in this primer are listed below.

- Place building as far from any secured perimeter as practical.
- Secure the perimeter against vehicular intrusion using landscaping or barrier methods.
- Use lightweight nonstructural elements on the building exterior and interior.
- Place unsecured areas exterior to the main structure or in the exterior bay.
- Incorporate measures to resist progressive collapse.
- Design exterior window systems and cladding so that the framing, connections, and supporting structure have a lateral-load-resistance that is equal to or higher than the transparency or panel.
- Place air intakes as far above the ground level as practical.
- Physically isolate vulnerable areas such as the entries and delivery areas from the rest of the structure by using floor-to-floor walls in these areas.
- Use redundant, separated mechanical/electrical control systems.

1.2 CONTENTS AND ORGANIZATION OF THE REPORT

This report provides basic qualitative and descriptive information characterizing potential terrorist threats: the effects of terrorist-caused explosions or releases of chemical, biological, and radiological (CBR) agents; and measures that can be taken to limit and mitigate their impacts on buildings and their occupants.

Because explosive attacks are expected to remain the dominant terrorist threat, most of the guidance in the document relates to explosions and limiting their effects. In addition to descriptive information and guidance, each chapter identifies references for further reading. Chapter 2 focuses principally on bomb (explosion) threats, likely targets, and likelihood of occurrence. Weapons effects are described in Chapter 3, which discusses blast pressure waves, initial blast forces, and the decay of these forces with time and distance. Chapter 4 focuses on damage caused by explosions, including damage mechanisms for various building elements and systems, including both structural and nonstructural components. Topics include (1) progressive collapse, (2) comparisons with forces imposed by other extreme loads, such as earthquakes and wind storms, and (3) the potential extent and distribution of deaths and injuries resulting from various damage mechanisms. Design approaches to limit or mitigate damage caused by bomb attacks are described in Chapter 5. Goals include preventing collapse (at least until the building can be fully evacuated) and reducing the effects of flying debris. Security measures described include: (1) preventing an attack, (2) delaying an attack, and (3) mitigating the effects of these attacks.

The heart of the document is Chapter 6, which contains extensive qualitative design guidance for limiting or mitigating the effects of terrorist attacks, focusing primarily on explosions, but also addressing chemical, biological, and radiological attacks. Checklists of mitigation measures are provided at the end of each major section. Site and layout design guidance is provided in Section 6.1. Important concepts are stand-off distance from the perimeter property line, controlled access zones, and anti-ram barriers, which can be either passive or active. Section 6.2 describes architectural issues and attributes affecting the impact of explosions on buildings. The primary focus is on building shape, placement, exterior ornamentation, and the functional layout of the interior. Structural design issues are discussed in Section 6.3. Topics include (1) methods to prevent progressive collapse; (2) the selection of a building structural system, including desirable attributes of the system; (3) structural layout (the placement of structural elements); (4) design methods, including the relationship between security design and design for conventional loads; and (5) the design of critical structural elements, focusing on the exterior frame, roof system, floor system, interior columns, and interior walls. Section 6.4 addresses the building envelope; i.e., exterior walls and cladding, window systems, and other openings. Specific guidance is provided on exterior wall and cladding design. Window design is given special consideration, including glass design, mullion design, and frame and anchorage design. Guidance is also given on wall design, multi-hazard considerations, and the design of other openings (doors and louvers). Issues relating to the design and placement of mechanical and electrical systems are described in Section 6.5. Topics addressed include emergency egress routes, air intakes, emergency power systems, fuel storage, ventilation systems, the fire-control center, emergency elevators, the smoke and fire detection and alarm systems, the sprinkler and standpipe system, smoke-control systems, and the communication system. Finally, Section 6.6 addresses issues specific to chemical, biological, and radiological protection. Issues discussed include air intakes, mechanical areas, return air systems, vulnerable internal areas (lobbies, loading docks, and mail sorting areas), zoning of HVAC systems, positive pressurization, air-tightness, filtration systems, detection systems, management of emergency response using the fire/HVAC control center, and evolving technologies for CBR prevention.

Chapter 7 discusses special considerations for multi-family residential buildings, buildings that include retail uses, and light-industrial buildings. Chapter 8 discusses cost issues, including some general suggestions on prioritizing potential security enhancements.

1.3 FURTHER READING

Other recently issued FEMA documents related to man-made hazards are listed below.

Federal Emergency Management Agency, FEMA 426, *Reference Manual to Mitigate Potential Terrorist Attacks Against Buildings.*

Federal Emergency Management Agency, FEMA 428, *Primer for Designing Safe School Projects in Case of Terrorist Attacks.*

Federal Emergency Management Agency, FEMA 429*, Primer for Terrorist Risk Reduction in High Occupancy Buildings.*

Federal Emergency Management Agency, FEMA 430, *Security Component for Architectural Design.*

TERRORIST THREATS 2

2.1 OVERVIEW OF POSSIBLE THREATS

This primer addresses several types of terrorist threats, which are listed below.

Explosive Threats:

- Vehicle weapon
- Hand-delivered weapon

Airborne Chemical, Biological, and Radiological Threats:

- Large-scale, external, air-borne release
- External release targeting building
- Internal release

Although it is possible that the dominant threat mode may change in the future, bombings have historically been a favorite tactic of terrorists. Ingredients for homemade bombs are easily obtained on the open market, as are the techniques for making bombs. Bombings are easy and quick to execute. Finally, the dramatic component of explosions in terms of the sheer destruction they cause creates a media sensation that is highly effective in transmitting the terrorist's message to the public.

2.2 EXPLOSIVE ATTACKS

From the standpoint of structural design, the vehicle bomb is the most important consideration. Vehicle bombs are able to deliver a sufficiently large quantity of explosives to cause potentially devastating structural damage. Security design intended to limit or mitigate damage from a vehicle bomb assumes that the bomb is detonated at a so-called critical location(see Figure 2-1). The critical location is a function of the site, the building layout, and the security measures in place. For a vehicle bomb, the critical location is taken to be at the closest point that a vehicle can approach, assuming that all security measures are in place. This may be a parking area directly beneath the occupied building, the loading dock, the curb directly outside the facility, or at a vehicle-access control gate where inspection takes place, depending on the level of protection incorporated into the design.

Another explosive attack threat is the small bomb that is hand delivered. Small weapons can cause the greatest damage when brought into vulnerable, unsecured areas of the building interior, such as the build-

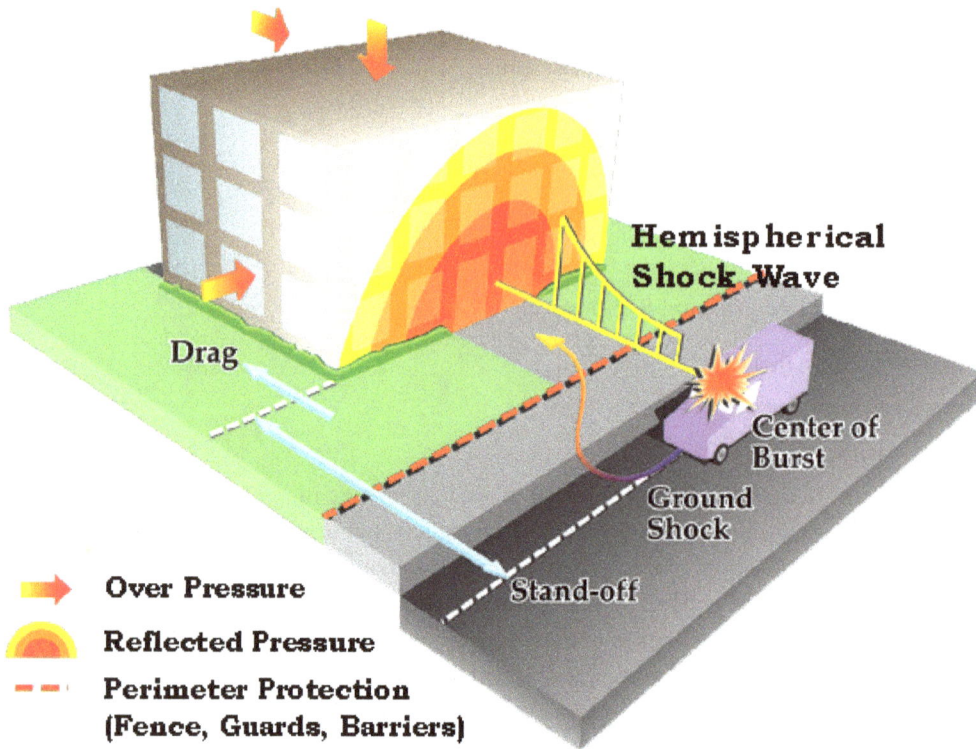

Over Pressure

Reflected Pressure

Perimeter Protection (Fence, Guards, Barriers)

Figure 2-1   Schematic of vehicle weapon threat parameters and definitions

ing lobby, mail room, and retail spaces. Recent events around the world make it clear that there is an increased likelihood that bombs will be delivered by persons who are willing to sacrifice their own lives. Hand-carried explosives are typically on the order of five to ten pounds of TNT equivalent. However, larger charge weights, in the 50 to 100 pounds TNT equivalent range, can be readily carried in rolling cases. Mail bombs are typically less than ten pounds of TNT equivalent.

In general, the largest credible explosive size is a function of the security measures in place. Each line of security may be thought of as a sieve, reducing the size of the weapon that may gain access. Therefore the largest weapons are considered in totally unsecured public space (e.g., in a vehicle on the nearest public street), and the smallest weapons are considered in the most secured areas of the building (e.g., in a briefcase smuggled past the screening station).

Two parameters define the design threat: the weapon size, measured in equivalent pounds of TNT, and the standoff. The standoff is the distance measured from the center of gravity of the charge to the component of interest.

The design weapon size is usually selected by the owner in collaboration with security and protective design consultants (i.e., engineers who specialize in the design of structures to mitigate the effects of explosions). Although there are few unclassified sources giving the sizes of weapons that have been used in previous attacks throughout the world, security consultants have valuable information that may be used to evaluate the range of charge weights that might be reasonably considered for the intended occupancy. Security consultants draw upon the experience of other countries such as Great Britain and Israel where terrorist attacks have been more prevalent, as well as data gathered by U.S. sources.

To put the weapon size into perspective, it should be noted that thousands of deliberate explosions occur every year within the United States, but the vast majority of them have weapon yields less than five pounds. The number of large-scale vehicle weapon attacks that have used hundreds of pounds of TNT during the past twenty years is by comparison very small.

The design vehicle weapon size will usually be much smaller than the largest credible threat. The design weapon size is typically measured in hundreds of pounds rather than thousands of pounds of TNT equivalent. The decision is usually based on a trade-off between the largest credible attack directed against the building and the design constraints of the project. Further, it is common for the design pressures and impulses to be less than the actual peak pressures and impulses acting on the building. This is the approach that the federal government has taken in their design criteria for federally owned domestic office buildings. There are several reasons for this choice.

1. The likely target is often not the building under design, but a high-risk building that is nearby. Historically, more building damage has been due to collateral effects than direct attack.

2. It is difficult to quantify the risk of man-made hazards. However, qualitatively it may be stated that the chance of a large-scale terrorist attack occurring is extremely low. A smaller explosive attack is far more likely.

3. Providing a level of protection that is consistent with standards adopted for federal office buildings enhances opportunities for leas-

ing to government agencies in addition to providing a clear statement regarding the building's safety to other potential tenants.

4. The added robustness inherent in designing for a vehicle bomb of moderate size will improve the performance of the building under all explosion scenarios.

2.3 FURTHER READING

Technical Support Working Group, ___, *Terrorist Bomb Threat Stand-Off Card with Explanation of Use*, Technical Support Working Group, Washington, D.C. http://www.tswg.gov/tswg/prods_pubs/newBTSCPress.htm

U.S. Department of the Treasury / Bureau of Alcohol, Tobacco and Firearms, 1999, *Vehicle Bomb Explosion Hazard And Evacuation Distance Tables*, Department of the Treasury, Washington, D.C. (Request in writing, address information available at http://www.atf.treas.gov/pub/fire-explo_pub/i54001.htm

Federal Bureau of Investigation, 1999, *Terrorism in the United States,* U.S. Department of Justice, Federal Bureau of Investigation, Counterterrorism Division, Washington, DC. http://www.fbi.gov/publications/terror/terror99.pdf

The U.S. Department of State, 2002, *Patterns of Global Terrorism 2001.* The U.S. Department of State, Washington, DC. http://www.state.gov/s/ct/rls/pgtrpt/2001/pdf/

WEAPONS EFFECTS   3

3.1   DESCRIPTION OF EXPLOSION FORCES

An explosion is an extremely rapid release of energy in the form of
light, heat, sound, and a shock wave. The shock wave consists of highly
compressed air that wave-reflects off the ground surface to produce a
hemispherical propagation of the wave that travels outward from the
source at supersonic velocities (see Figure 2-1). As the shock wave
expands, the incident or over-pressures decrease. When it encounters a
surface that is in line-of-sight of the explosion, the wave is reflected,
resulting in a tremendous amplification of pressure. Unlike acoustical
waves, which reflect with an amplification factor of two, shock waves can
reflect with an amplification factor of up to thirteen, due to the supersonic velocity of the shock wave at impact. The magnitude of the reflec-
tion factor is a function of the proximity of the explosion and the angle
of incidence of the shock wave on the surface.

The pressures decay rapidly with time (i.e., exponentially), measured
typically in thousandths of a second (milliseconds). Diffraction effects,
caused by building features such as re-entrant corners and overhangs of
the building may act to confine the air blast, prolonging its duration.
Late in the explosive event, the shock wave becomes negative, followed
by a partial vacuum, which creates suction behind the shock wave(see
Figure 3-1). Immediately following the vacuum, air rushes in, creating a
powerful wind or drag pressure on all surfaces of the building. This
wind picks up and carries flying debris in the vicinity of the detonation.
In an external explosion, a portion of the energy is also imparted to the
ground, creating a crater and generating a ground shock wave analo-
gous to a high-intensity, short-duration earthquake.

The peak pressure is a function of the weapon size or yield, and the
cube of the distance (see Figure 3-2). For an explosive threat defined by
its charge weight and standoff, the peak incident and reflected pressures of the shock wave and other useful parameters such as the incident and reflected impulse, shock velocity, and time of arrival are
evaluated using charts available in military handbooks.

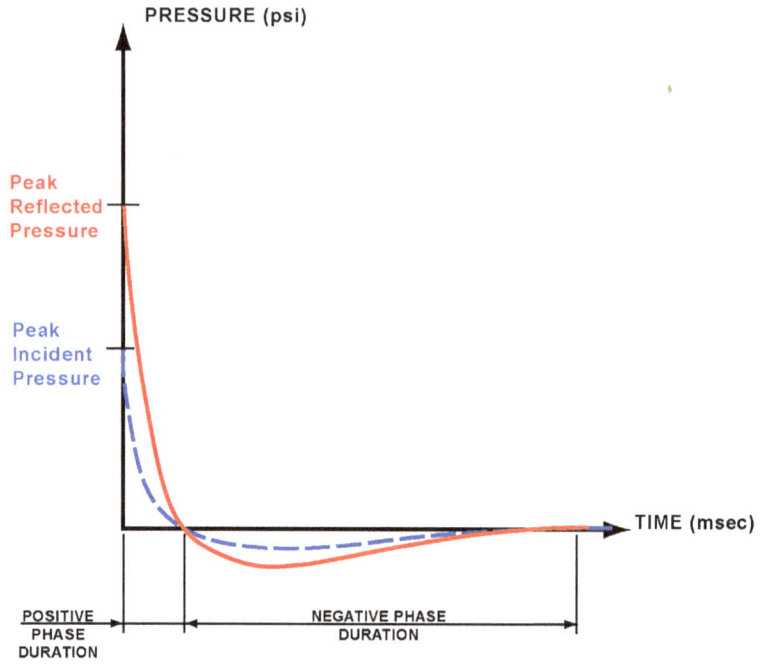

Figure 3-1   Air-blast pressure time history

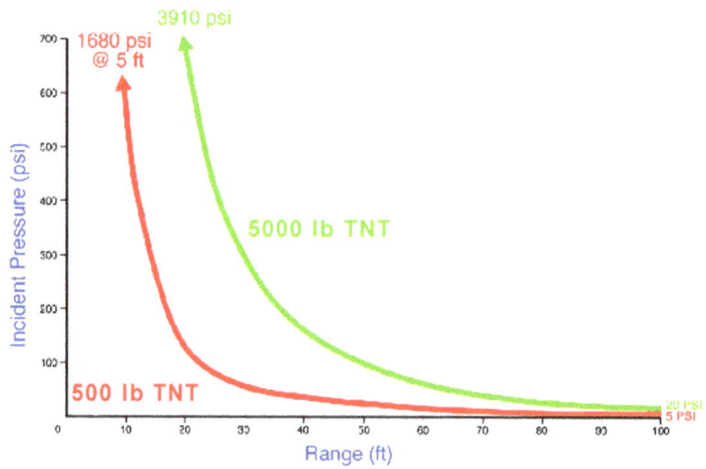

Figure 3-2   Plots showing pressure decay with distance

3.2 FURTHER READING

These references provide charts for evaluating explosive loads as well as extensive information regarding the structural design of buildings to resist explosive attack.

U.S. Air Force, 1989, *ESL-TR-87-57, Protective Construction Design Manual*, Contact Airbus Technologies Division (AFRL/MLQ) at Tyndall Air Force Base, Florida, via e-mail to techinfo@afrl.af.mil. [Superseded by Army Technical Manual TM 5-855-1 (Air Force Pamphlet AFPAM 32-1147(I), Navy Manual NAVFAC P-1080, DSWA Manual DAH-SCWEMAN-97), December 1997]

U.S. Army Corps of Engineers, 1990, TM 5-1300, *Structures to Resist Accidental Explosions*, U.S. Army Corps of Engineers, Washington, D.C., (also Navy NAVFAC (Naval Facilities) P-397, Air Force Regulation 88-2); Contact David Hyde, U.S. Army Engineer Research and Development Center, 3909 Halls Ferry Road, Vicksburg, Mississippi 39180 or via e-mail to hyded@ex1.wes.army.mil

U.S. Department of Energy, 1992, DOE/TIC 11268, *A Manual for the Prediction of Blast and Fragment Loadings on Structures*, Southwest Research Institute, Albuquerque, New Mexico.

4.1   PREDICTING DAMAGE LEVELS

The extent and severity of damage and injuries in an explosive event cannot be predicted with perfect certainty. Past events show that the specifics of the failure sequence for an individual building due to air-blast effects and debris impact significantly affect the overall level of damage.

For instance, two adjacent columns of a building may be roughly the same distance from the explosion, but only one fails because it is struck by a fragment in a particular way that initiates collapse. The other, by chance, is not struck and remains in place. Similarly, glass failures may occur outside of the predicted areas due to air-blast diffraction effects caused by the arrangement of buildings and their heights in the vicinity of the explosion. The details of the physical setting surrounding a particular occupant may greatly influence the level of injury incurred. The position of the person, seated or standing, facing towards or away from the event as it happens, may result in injuries ranging from minor to severe.

Despite these uncertainties, it is possible to calculate the expected extent of damage and injuries to be expected in an explosive event, based on the size of the explosion, distance from the event, and assumptions about the construction of the building. Additionally, there is strong evidence to support a relationship between injury patterns and structural damage patterns.

4.2   DAMAGE MECHANISMS

Damage due to the air-blast shock wave may be divided into direct air-blast effects and progressive collapse.

Direct air-blast effects are damage caused by the high-intensity pressures of the air blast close to the explosion. These may induce localized failure of exterior walls, windows, roof systems, floor systems, and columns.

Progressive collapse refers to the spread of an initial local failure from element to element, eventually resulting in a disproportionate extent of collapse relative to the zone of initial damage. Localized damage due to direct air-blast effects may or may not progress, depending on the design and construction of the building. To produce a progressive collapse, the weapon must be in close proximity to a critical load-bearing element. Progressive collapse can propagate vertically upward or downward (e.g., Ronan Point[1]) from the source of the explosion, and it can propagate laterally from bay to bay as well.

The pressures that an explosion exerts on building surfaces may be several orders of magnitude greater than the loads for which the building is designed. The shock wave also acts in directions that the building may not have been designed for, such as upward pressure on the floor system. In terms of sequence of response, the air blast first impinges the exterior envelope of the building. The pressure wave pushes on the exterior walls and may cause wall failure and window breakage. As the shock wave continues to expand, it enters the structure, pushing both upward on the ceilings and downward on the floors (see Figure 4-1).

Floor failure is common in large-scale vehicle-delivered explosive attacks, because floor slabs typically have a large surface area for the pressure to act on and a comparably small thickness. Floor failure is particularly common for close-in and internal explosions. The loss of a floor system increases the unbraced height of the supporting columns, which may lead to structural instability.

For hand-carried weapons that are brought into the building and placed on the floor away from a primary vertical load-bearing element, the response will be more localized with damage and injuries extending a bay or two in each direction (see Figure 4-2). Although the weapon is smaller, the air-blast effects are amplified due to multiple reflections from interior surfaces. Typical damage types that may be expected include:

○ localized failure of the floor system immediately below the weapon;

○ damage and possible localized failure for the floor system above the weapon;

○ damage and possible localized failure of nearby concrete and masonry walls;

○ failure of nonstructural elements such as partition walls, false ceilings, ductwork, window treatments; and

1. "Ronan Point" is the name of a high-rise pre-cast housing complex in Britain that suffered progressive collapse in 1968 due to a gas explosion in a kitchen in a corner bay of the building. The explosion caused the collapse of all corner bays below it and was a seminal event for progressive collapse, precipitating funding for research and development in the United States, Britain and Europe. As a result, Britain developed a set of implicit design requirements to resist progressive collapse in buildings and, in the 1970s, the National Institute of Standards and Technology (NIST) produced some state-of-the-practice reports on this topic.

BUILDING DAMAGE

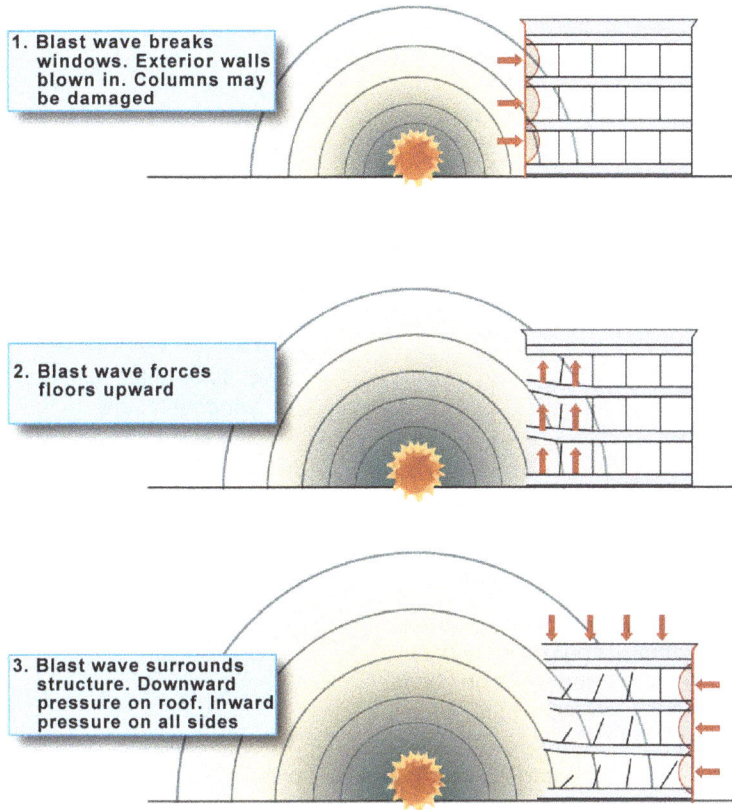

1. Blast wave breaks windows. Exterior walls blown in. Columns may be damaged

2. Blast wave forces floors upward

3. Blast wave surrounds structure. Downward pressure on roof. Inward pressure on all sides

Figure 4-1   Schematic showing sequence of building damage due to a vehicle weapon

○ flying debris generated by furniture, computer equipment, and other contents.

More extensive damage, possibly leading to progressive collapse, may occur if the weapon is strategically placed directly against a primary load-bearing element such as a column.

In comparison to other hazards such as earthquake or wind, an explosive attack has several distinguishing features, listed below.

○ *The intensity of the localized pressures acting on building components can be several orders of magnitude greater than these other hazards.* It is not uncommon for the peak pressure on the building from a vehicle weapon parked along the curb to be in excess of 100 psi.   Major damage and failure of building components is expected even for relatively small weapons, in close proximity to the building.

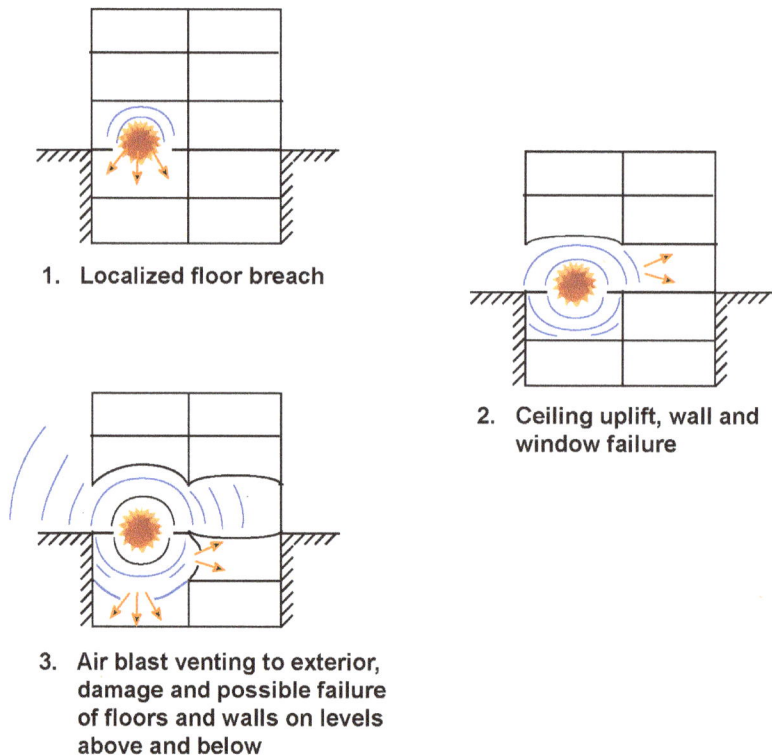

1. Localized floor breach

2. Ceiling uplift, wall and window failure

3. Air blast venting to exterior, damage and possible failure of floors and walls on levels above and below

Figure 4-2   Schematics showing sequence of building damage due to a package weapon

○ *Explosive pressures decay extremely rapidly with distance from the source.* Pressures acting on the building, particularly on the side facing the explosion, may vary significantly, causing a wide range of damage types. As a result, air blast tends to cause more localized damage than other hazards that have a more global effect.

○ *The duration of the event is very short, measured in thousandths of a second, (milliseconds).* In terms of timing, the building is engulfed by the shockwave and direct air-blast damage occurs within tens to hundreds of milliseconds from the time of detonation due to the supersonic velocity of the shock wave and the nearly instantaneous response of the structural elements. By comparison, earthquake events last for seconds and wind loads may act on the building for minutes or longer.

BUILDING DAMAGE

4.3 CORRELATION BETWEEN DAMAGE AND INJURIES

Three types of building damage can lead to injuries and possible fatalities. The most severe building response is collapse. In past incidents, collapse has caused the most extensive fatalities. For the Oklahoma City bombing in 1995 (see Figure 4-3), nearly 90 percent of the building occupants who lost their lives were in the collapsed portion of the Alfred P. Murrah Federal Office Building. Many of the survivors in the collapsed region were on the lower floors and had been trapped in void spaces under concrete slabs.

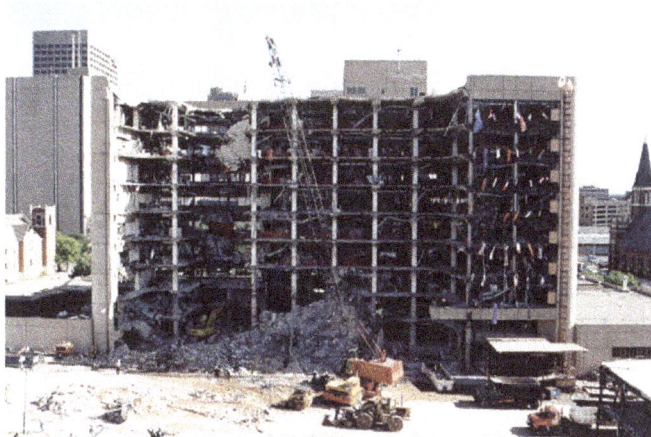

Figure 4-3   Exterior view of Alfred P. Murrah Federal Building collapse

Although the targeted building is at greatest risk of collapse, other nearby buildings may also collapse. For instance, in the Oklahoma City bombing, a total of nine buildings collapsed. Most of these were unreinforced masonry structures that fortunately were largely unoccupied at the time of the attack. In the bombing of the U.S. embassy in Nairobi, Kenya in 1998, the collapse of the Uffundi building, a concrete building adjacent to the embassy, caused hundreds of fatalities.

For buildings that remain standing, the next most severe type of injury-producing damage is flying debris generated by exterior cladding. Depending on the severity of the incident, fatalities may occur as a result of flying structural debris. Some examples of exterior wall failure causing injuries are listed below.

○ In the Oklahoma City bombing, several persons lost their lives after being struck by structural debris generated by infill walls of a concrete frame building in the Water Resources building across the street from the Murrah building.

○ In the Khobar Towers bombing in 1996 (see Figure 4-4), most of the 19 U.S. servicemen who loss their lives were impacted by high-velocity projectiles created by the failed exterior cladding on the wall that faced the weapon. The building was an all-precast, reinforced concrete structure with robust connections between the slabs and walls. The numerous lines of vertical support along with the ample lateral stability provided by the "egg crate" configuration of the structural system prevented collapse.

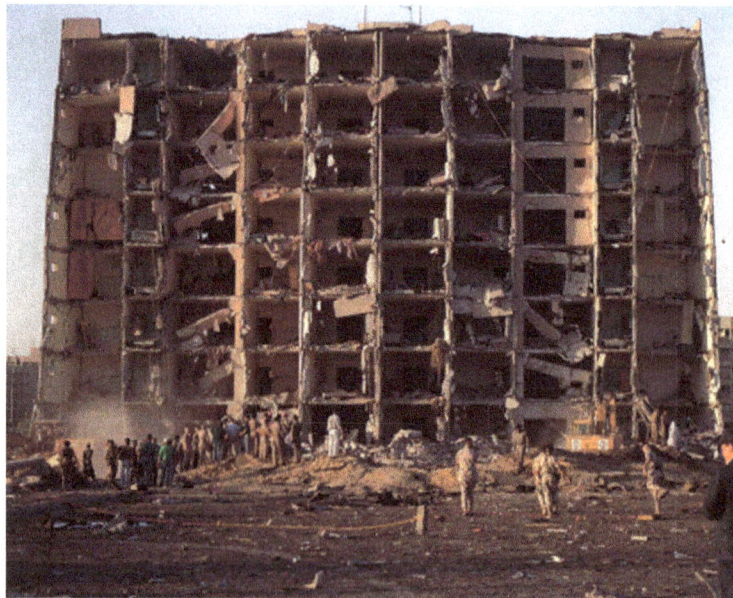

Figure 4-4   Exterior view of Khobar Towers exterior wall failure

○ In the bombing of the U.S. embassy in Dar es Salaam, Tanzania in 1998, the exterior unreinforced masonry infill wall of the concrete-framed embassy building blew inward. The massiveness of the construction generated relatively low-velocity projectiles that injured and partially buried occupants, but did not cause fatalities.

Even if the building remains standing and no structural damage occurs, extensive injuries can occur due to nonstructural damage (see

Figure 4-5). Typically, for large-scale incidents, these types of injuries occur to persons who are in buildings that are within several blocks of the incident. Although these injuries are often not life-threatening, many people can be affected, which has an impact on the ability of local medical resources to adequately respond. An example of nonstructural damage causing injuries is the extensive glass lacerations that occurred in the Oklahoma City Bombing within the Regency Towers apartment building, which was approximately 500 feet from the Murrah Building. In this incident, glass laceration injuries extended as far as 10 blocks from the bombing. Another example is the bombing of the U.S. embassy in Nairobi, Kenya. The explosion occurred near one of the major intersections of the city, which was heavily populated at the time of the bombing, causing extensive glass lacerations to passersby. The ambassador, who was attending a meeting at an office building across from the embassy, sustained an eye injury as a result of extensive window failure in the building.

A summary of the relationship between the type of damage and the resulting injuries is given in Table 4-1.

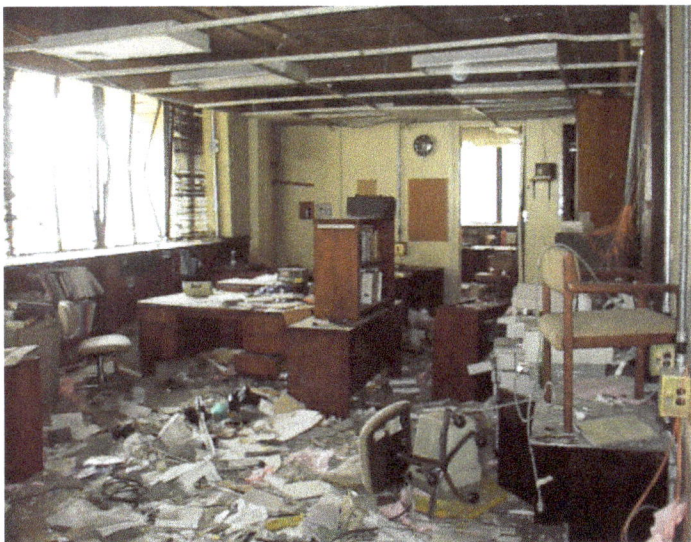

Figure 4-5   Photograph showing non-structural damage in building impacted by blast

Table 4-1: Damage and Injuries due to Explosion Effects

Distance from Explosion	Most Severe Building Damage Expected	Associated Injuries
Close-in	General Collapse	Fatality due impact and crushing
Moderate	Exterior wall failure, exterior bay floor slab damage	Skull fracture, concussion
Far	Window breakage, falling light fixtures, flying debris	Lacerations from flying glass, abrasions from being thrown against objects or objects striking occupants

4.4 FURTHER READING

Federal Emergency Management Agency, 1996, FEMA 277. *The Oklahoma City Bombing: Improving Building Performance through Multi-Hazard Mitigation*, Federal Emergency Management Agency Washington, D.C. http://www.fema.gov/mit/bpat/bpat009.htm

Federal Emergency Management Agency, 2002, FEMA 403. *World Trade Center Building Performance Study: Data Collection, Preliminary Observations, and Recommendations.* Federal Emergency Management Agency, Washington, D.C. http://www.fema.gov/library/wtc-study.shtm

Hinman, E. and Hammond, D., 1997, *Lessons from the Oklahoma City Bombing: Defensive Design Techniques.* American Society of Civil Engineers (ASCE Press), Reston, VA. http://www.asce.org/publications/booksdisplay.cfm?type=9702295

The House National Security Committee, 1996. *Statement of Chairman Floyd D. Spence on the Report of the Bombing of Khobar Towers.* The House National Security Committee, Washington, DC. http://www.house.gov/hasc/Publications/104thCongress/Reports/saudi.pdf

U.S. Department of State, 1999. *The Report of the Accountability Review Board on the Embassy Bombings in Nairobi and Dar es Salaam on August 7, 1998.* Department of State, Washington, DC. http://www.state.gov/www/regions/africa/accountability_report.html

Mallonee, S., Shariat, S., Stennies, G., Waxweiler, R., Hogan, D., & Jordan, F., 1996, Physical injuries and fatalities resulting from the Oklahoma City bombing. *The Journal of the American Medical Association*, Vol. 276 No. 5: pages 382-387. http://jama.ama-assn.org/cgi/con-

tent/abstract/276/5/382?max-
toshow=&HITS=10&hits=10&RESULTFORMAT=&fulltext=oklaho
ma+city+bomb-
ing&searchid=1048882533579_3224&stored_search=&FIRSTIN-
DEX=0

5.1 GOALS OF THE DESIGN APPROACH

It is impractical to design a civilian structure to remain undamaged from a large explosion. The protective objectives are therefore related to the type of building and its function. For an office, retail, residential, or light industrial building, where the primary asset is the occupants, the objective is to minimize loss of life. Because of the severity of large scale explosion incidents, the goals are by necessity modest. Moreover, it is recognized that the building will be unusable after the event. This approach is considered a damage-limiting or damage-mitigating approach to design.

To save lives, the primary goals of the design professional are to reduce building damage and to prevent progressive collapse of the building, at least until it can be fully evacuated. A secondary goal is to maintain emergency functions until evacuation is complete.

The design professional is able to reduce building damage by incorporating access controls that allow building security to keep large threats away from the building and to limit charge weights that can be brought into the building.

Preventing the building from collapsing is the most important objective. Historically, the majority of fatalities that occur in terrorist attacks directed against buildings are due to building collapse. Collapse prevention begins with awareness by architects and engineers that structural integrity against collapse is important enough to be routinely considered in design. Features to improve general structural resistance to collapse can be incorporated into common buildings at affordable cost. At a higher level, designing the building to prevent progressive collapse can be accomplished by the alternate-path method (i.e., design for the building to remain standing following the removal of specific elements) or by direct design of components for air-blast loading.

Furthermore, building design may be optimized by facilitating evacuation, rescue, and recovery efforts through effective placement, structural design, and redundancy of emergency exits and critical mechanical/electrical systems. Through effective structural design, the overall damage levels may be reduced to make it easier it is for occupants to get out and emergency responders to safely enter.

Beyond the issues of preventing collapse, and facilitating evacuation/rescue the objective is to reduce flying debris generated by failed exterior walls, windows and other components to reduce the severity of injuries and the risk of fatalities. This may be accomplished through selection of appropriate materials and use of capacity-design methods to proportion elements and connections. A well designed system will provide predictable damage modes, selected to minimize injuries. Finally, good anti-terrorist design is a multidisciplinary effort requiring the concerted efforts of the architect, structural engineer, security professional, and the other design team members. It is also critical for security design to be incorporated as early as possible in the design process to ensure a cost-effective, attractive solution.

5.2 SECURITY PRINCIPLES

This section provides some fundamental security concepts that place physical security into the context of overall facility security. The components of security include deception, intelligence, operational protection, and structural hardening. These components are interrelated (see Figure 5-1).

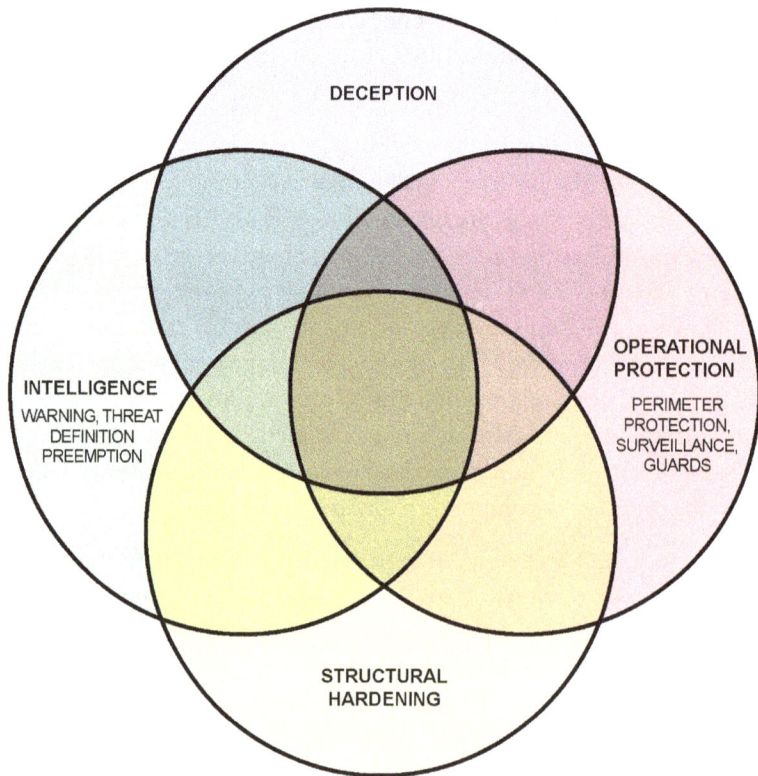

Figure 5-1   Components of security

Ideally, a potential terrorist attack is prevented or pre-empted through intelligence measures. If the attack does occur, physical security measures combine with operational forces (e.g., surveillance, guards, and sensors) to provide layers of defense that delay and/or thwart the attack. Deception may be used to make the facility appear to be a more protected or lower-risk facility than it actually is, thereby making it appear to be a less attractive target. Deception can also be used to misdirect the attacker to a portion of the facility that is non-critical. As a last resort, structural hardening is provided to save lives and facilitate evacuation and rescue by preventing building collapse and limiting flying debris.

Because of the interrelationship between physical and operational security measures, it is imperative for the owner and security professional to define early in the design process what extent of operational security is planned for various threat levels.

If properly implemented, physical security measures will contribute toward the goals listed below in prioritized order.

○ *Preventing an attack.* By making it more difficult to implement some of the more obvious attack scenarios (such as a parked car in the street) or making the target appear to be of low value in terms of the amount of sensation that would be generated if it were attacked, the would-be attacker may become discouraged from targeting the building. On the other hand, it may not be advantageous to make the facility too obviously protected or not protected, for this may have the opposite of the intended affect and provide an incentive to attack the building.

○ *Delaying the attack.* If an attack is initiated, properly designed landscape or architectural features can delay its execution by making it more difficult for the attacker to reach the intended target. This will give the security forces and authorities time to mobilize and possibly to stop the attack before it is executed. This is done by creating a buffer zone between the publicly accessible areas and the vital areas of the facility by means of an obstacle course, a serpentine path and/or a division of functions within the facility. Alternatively, through effective design, the attacker could be enticed to a non-critical part of the facility, thereby delaying the attack.

○ *Mitigating the effects of the attack.* If these precautions are implemented and the attack still takes place, then structural protection efforts will serve to control the extent and consequences of damage. In the context of the overall security provided to the building, structural protection is a last resort that only becomes effective after all other efforts to stop the attack have failed. In the event of an attack, the benefits of enhancements to life-safety systems may be realized in lives saved.

An effective way to implement these goals is to create layers of security within the facility (see Figure 5-2). The outermost layer is the perimeter

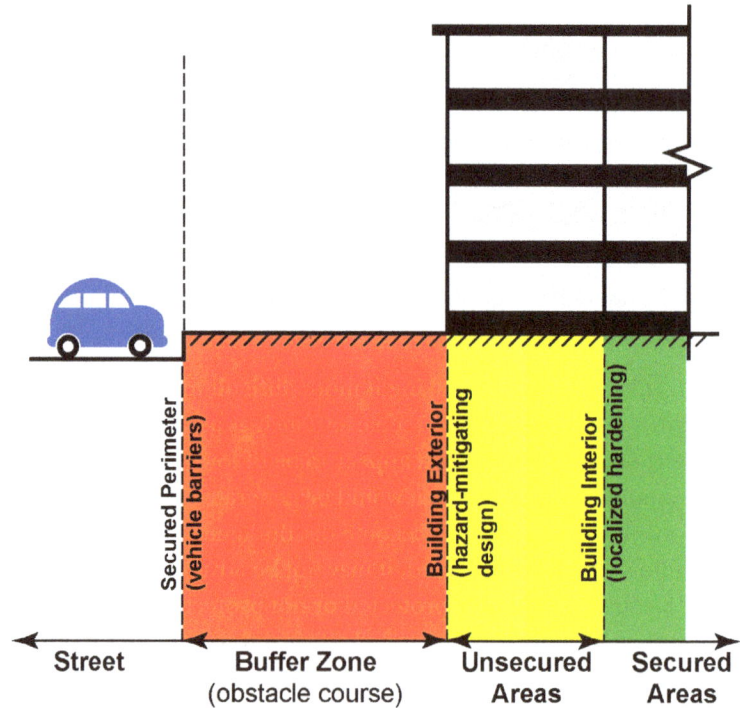

Figure 5-2   Schematic showing lines of defense against blast

of the facility. Interior to this line is the approach zone to the facility, then the building exterior, and finally the building interior. The interior of the building may be divided into successively more protected zones, starting with publicly accessible areas such as the lobby and retail space, to the more private areas of offices, and finally the vital functions such as the control room and emergency functions. The advantage of this approach is that once a line of protection is breached, the facility has not been completely compromised. Having multiple lines of defense provides redundancy to the security system, adding robustness to the design. Also, by using this approach, not all of the focus is on the outer layer of protection, which may lead to an unattractive, fortress-like appearance.

To provide a reliable design, each ring must have a uniform level of security provided along its entire length; security is only as strong as the weakest link.

To have a balanced design, both physical and operational security measures need to be implemented in the facility. Architects and engineers can contribute to an effective physical security system, which augments and facilitates the operational security functions. If security measures are left as an afterthought, expensive, unattractive, and make-shift security posts are the inevitable result. For more information on security, refer to FEMA 426 (*Reference Manual to Mitigate Potential Terrorist Attacks in High-Occupancy Buildings*).

5.3   FURTHER READING

Listed below are sources for some of the existing protective design criteria prepared by the federal government using the damage-limiting approach.

Federal Aviation Administration, 2001, *Recommended Security Guidelines for Airport Planning, Design and Construction* (DOT/FAA/AR-00/52), Associate Administrator for Civil Aviation Security Office of Civil Aviation Security, Policy and Planning, Federal Aviation Administration, Washington, D.C.

Interagency Security Committee. 2001, *Security Design Criteria for New Federal Office Buildings and Major Modernization Projects*, Washington D.C. [For Official Use Only] *http://www.oca.gsa.gov/restricted/protectedfiles/ISCCriteriaMay282001.PDF*

U.S. Department of Defense, 2002, *DoD Minimum Antiterrorism Standards for Buildings*. Unified Facilities Criteria (UFC), UFC 4-010-01, Department of Defense, Washington, D.C. *http://www.tisp.org/puglication/pubdetails.cfm?&pubID=105*

U.S. Department of State, Bureau of Diplomatic Security, *Architectural Engineering Design Guidelines* (5 Volumes) [For Official Use Only]

In this chapter, design guidance is provided for limiting or mitigating the effects of terrorist attacks. Guidance is provided for each of the following aspects of design: site location and layout, architectural, structural, building envelope, and mechanical and electrical systems. Sections 6.1 through 6.5 pertain to attack using explosive weapons. Protective measures against chemical, biological, and radiological attacks are discussed in Section 6.6. In each section, design guidance is discussed and recommendations are given for enhancing life safety.

> **Sections at a glance:**
>
> 6.1   Site location and Layout
> 6.2   Architectural
> 6.3   Structural
> 6.4   Building Envelope
> 6.5   Mechanical and Electrical Systems
> 6.6   Chemical, Biological, and Radiological Protection

6.1   SITE LOCATION AND LAYOUT

Because air-blast pressures decrease rapidly with distance, one of the most effective means of protecting assets is to increase the distance between a potential bomb and the assets to be protected. The best way to do this is to provide a continuous line of security along the perimeter of the facility to protect it from unscreened vehicles and to keep all vehicles as far away from critical assets as possible.

This section discusses the perimeter and the approach to the building. For discussion about building shape and placement on the site, see Section 6.2, Architectural.

6.1.1   Perimeter Line

The perimeter line of protection is the outermost line that can be protected by facility security measures. The perimeter needs to be designed to prevent carriers of large-scale weapons from gaining access to the site. In design, it is assumed that all large-scale explosive weapons (i.e., car bombs or truck bombs) are outside this line of defense. This line is defended by both physical and operational security methods.

It is recommended that the perimeter line be located as far as is practical from the building exterior. Many times, vulnerable buildings are located in urban areas where site conditions are tight. In this case, the options are obviously limited. Often, the perimeter line can be pushed out to the edge of the sidewalk by means of bollards, planters, and other obstacles. To push this line even further outward, restricting or eliminating parking along the curb can be arranged with the local authorities, but this can be a difficult and time consuming effort. In some cases, eliminating loading zones and street/lane closings are an option.

6.1.2 Controlled Access Zones

Access control refers to points of controlled access to the facility through the perimeter line. The controlled access check or inspection points for vehicles require architectural features or barriers to maintain the defensible perimeter. Architects and engineers can accommodate these security functions by providing adequate design for these areas, which makes it difficult for a vehicle to crash onto the site.

Deterrence and delay are major attributes of the perimeter security design that should be consistent with the landscaping objectives, such as emphasizing the open nature characterizing high-population buildings. Since it is impossible to thwart all possible threats, the objective is to make it difficult to successfully execute the easiest attack scenarios such as a car bomb detonated along the curb, or a vehicle jumping the curb and ramming into the building prior to detonation.

If space is available between the perimeter line and the building exterior, much can be done to delay an intruder. Examples include terraced landscaping, fountains, statues, staircases, circular driveways, planters, trees, high-strength cables hidden in bushes and any number of other obstacles that make it difficult to rapidly reach the building. Though individually these features may not be able to stop a vehicle, in combination, they form a daunting obstacle course. Other ideas for implementing secure landscaping features may be found in texts on Crime Prevention Through Environmental Design (CPTED). These concepts are useful for slowing down traffic, improving surveillance, and site circulation.

On the sides of the building that are close to the curb, where landscaping solutions are limited, anti-ram barriers capable of stopping a vehicle on impact are recommended for high-risk buildings. Barrier design methods are discussed in more detail below.

The location of access points should be oblique to oncoming streets so that it is difficult for a vehicle to gain enough velocity to break through these access locations. If the site provides straight-on access to the building, some mitigation options include concrete medians in the street to slow vehicles or, for high-risk buildings, use of anti-ram barriers along the curb capable of withstanding the impact of high-velocity vehicles.

Place parking as far as practical from the building. Off-site parking is recommended for high-risk facilities vulnerable to terrorist attack. If on-site surface parking or underground parking is provided, take precautions such as limiting access to these areas only to the building occupants and/or having all vehicles inspected in areas close-in to the building. If an underground area is used for a high-risk building, the garage should be placed adjacent to the building under a plaza area rather than directly underneath the building. To the extent practical, limit the size of vehicle that is able to enter the garage by imposing physical barriers on vehicle height.

6.1.3   Physical Protective Barriers

There are two basic categories of perimeter anti-ram barriers; passive (or fixed) and active (or operable). Each is described below.

6.1.3.1   Passive Barriers

Passive barriers are those that are fixed in place and do not allow for vehicle entry. These are to be used away from vehicle access points. The majority of these are constructed in place.

For lower-risk buildings without straight-on vehicular access, it may be appropriate to install surface-mounted systems such as planters, or to use landscaping features to deter an intrusion threat. An example of a simple but effective landscaping solution is to install a deep permanent planter around the building with a wall that is as high as a car or truck bumper.

Individual planters mounted on the sidewalk resist impact through inertia and friction between the planter and the pavement. It can be expected that the planter will move as a result of the impact. For a successful design, the maximum displacement of the planter should be less than the setback distance to the building. The structure supporting the weight of the planter must be considered prior to installation.

To further reduce displacement, the planter may be placed several inches below the pavement surface. A roughened, grouted interface surface will also improve performance.

The traditional anti-ram solution entails the use of bollards (see Figure 6-1). Bollards are concrete-filled steel pipes that are placed every few feet along the curb of a sidewalk to prevent vehicle intrusion. In order for them to resist the impact of a vehicle, the bollard needs to be fully embedded into a concrete strip foundation that is several feet deep. The height of the bollard above ground should be higher than the bumper of the vehicle. The spacing of the bollards is based on several factors including ADA (American Disabilities Act) requirements, the minimum width of a vehicle, and the number of bollards required to resist the impact. As a rule of thumb, the center-to-center spacing

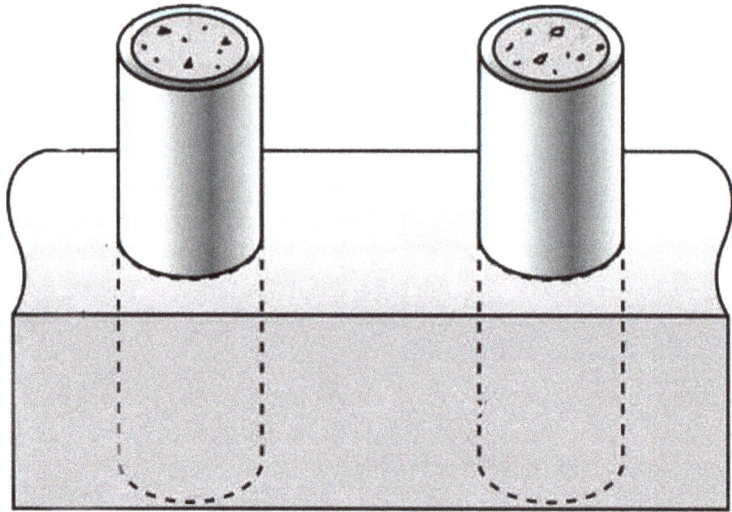

Figure 6-1   Schematic of typical anti-ram bollard

should be between three and five feet to be effective. The height of the bollard is to be at least as high as the bumper of the design threat vehicle, which is taken typically between two and three feet.

An alternative to a bollard is a plinth wall, which is a continuous knee wall constructed of reinforced concrete with a buried foundation (see Figure 6-2). The wall may be fashioned into a bench, a base for a fence, or the wall of a planter. To be effective, the height needs to be at least as high as the vehicle bumper.

For effectiveness, the barriers need to be placed as close to the curb as possible. However, the property line of buildings often does not extend to the curb. Therefore, to place barriers with foundations near the curb, a permit is required by the local authorities, which can be a difficult time-consuming effort to obtain. To avoid this, building owners are often inclined to place bollards along the property line, which significantly reduces the effectiveness of the barrier system.

The foundation of the bollard and plinth wall system can present challenges. There are sometimes vaults or basements below the pavement that extend to the property line, which often require special foundation details. Unless the foundation wall can sustain the reaction forces, significant damage may occur.

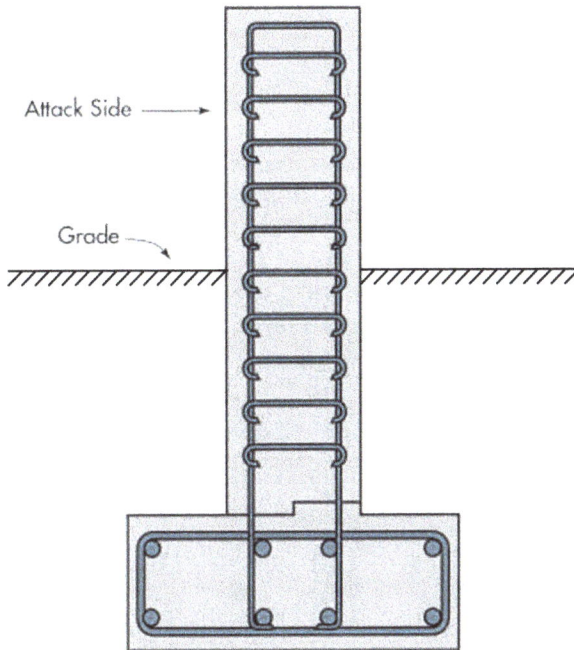

Figure 6-2   Schematic of typical anti-ram knee wall

Below-ground utilities that are frequently close to the pavement surface present additional problems. Their location may not be known with certainty, and this often leads to difficulties during construction. This also can be a strong deterrent to selecting barriers with foundations as a solution. However, for high-risk facilities, it is recommended that these issues be resolved during the design phase so that a reliable anti-ram barrier solution can be installed. For lower-risk buildings without straight-on vehicular access, it may be more appropriate to install surface-mounted systems such as planters or to use landscaping features to deter an intrusion threat. An example of a simple but effective landscaping solution is to install a deep permanent planter around the building with a wall that is at least as high as a car or truck bumper.

6.1.3.2   Active Systems

At vehicular access points, active or operational anti-ram systems are required. There are off-the-shelf products available that have been rated to resist various levels of car and truck impacts. Solutions include:

◯ crash beams;

- ○ crash gates;
- ○ surface-mounted plate systems;
- ○ retractable bollards; and
- ○ rotating-wedge systems.

The first three systems listed above generally have lower impact ratings than the last two listed. Check with the manufacturer to ensure that the system has been tested to meet the impact requirements for your project.

It is important that the installation of hydraulically operated systems be performed by a qualified contractor to ensure a reliable system that will work properly in all weather conditions.

6.1.4   Effectiveness of Anti-Ram Barriers

The effectiveness of an anti-ram barrier is based on the amount of energy it can absorb versus the amount of kinetic energy imparted by vehicle impact. The angle of approach reduces this energy in non-head-on situations, and the energy absorbed by the crushing of the vehicle also reduces the energy imparted to the barriers. The kinetic energy imparted to the wall is one-half the product of the vehicle mass and its impact velocity squared. Because the velocity term is squared, a change in velocity affects the energy level more than a change in vehicle weight. For this reason, it is important to review lines of approach to define areas where a vehicle has a long, straight road to pick up speed before impact.

The vehicle weight used for the design of barriers typically ranges from 4000 lb for cars up to 15,000 lb for trucks. Impact velocities typically range from 30 mph for oblique impact areas (i.e., where the oncoming street is parallel to the curb) up to 50 mph where there is straight-on access (i.e., where the oncoming street is perpendicular to the curb).

The kinetic energy of the vehicle at impact is absorbed by the barrier system. For fixed systems (like a concrete bollard), the energy is absorbed through the deformational strain energy absorbed by the barrier, soil, and the vehicle. For movable systems (like a surface-mounted planter) energy is absorbed through shear friction against the pavement and vehicle deformation.

Barrier effectiveness is ranked in terms of the amount of displacement of the system due to impact. Standard ratings defined by the federal government define the distance the vehicle travels before it is brought to rest. The most effective systems stop the vehicles within three feet, moderately effective barriers stop the vehicle within 20 feet, and the least effective systems require up to 50 feet.

6.1.5 Checklist – Site and Layout Design Guidance

✔ Provide a continuous line of defense around the site as far from the building as practical.

✔ Place vehicular access points away from oncoming streets.

✔ Limit the number of vehicular entrances through the secured perimeter line

✔ Use a series of landscape features to create an obstacle course between the building and the perimeter. This approach is most effective if used in areas where there is ample setback.

✔ Design planters for the design-level impact to displace the planter a distance less than the setback.

✔ Use anti-ram barriers along curbs, particularly on sides of the building that have a small setback and in areas where high-velocity impact is possible.

✔ Use operable anti-ram barriers at vehicular access points. Select barriers rated to provide the desired level of protection against the design impact.

6.1.6 Further Reading

National Capital Planning Commission, 2001. *Designing for Security in the Nation's Capital,* National Capital Planning Commission, Washington, D.C. http://www.ncpc.gov/whats_new/ITFreport.pdf

U.S. Air Force, 1997, *Installation Force Protection Guide,* Air Force Center for Environmental Excellence, Brooks Air Force Base, Texas http://www.afcee.brooks.af.mil/dc/dcd/arch/force.pdf

Crowe, T. D., 2000, *Crime Prevention Through Environmental Design: Applications Of Architectural Design And Space Management Concepts* (2nd Ed.), Butterworth-Heinemann, Stoneham, Massachusetts. ISBN: 075067198X http://www.amazon.com/exec/obidos/ASIN/075067198X/103-7416668-4182264#product-details

Newman, O., 1996, *Creating Defensible Space,* U.S. Department of Housing and Urban Development, Washington, D.C. http://www.huduser.org/publications/pdf/def.pdf

6.2 ARCHITECTURAL

There is much that can be done architecturally to mitigate the effects of a terrorist bombing on a facility. These measures often cost nothing or very little if implemented early in the design process. It is recommended that protective design and security consultants are used as early as possible in the design process. They should be involved in the site selection and their input should be sought during programming and schematic design.

6.2.1 Building Exterior

This section discusses the building shape, placement, and exterior ornamentation. For a discussion of exterior cladding, see Section 6.4, Building Envelope.

At the building exterior, the focus shifts from deterring and delaying the attack to mitigating the effects of an explosion. The exterior envelope of the building is most vulnerable to an exterior explosive threat because it is the part of the building closest to the weapon, and it is typically built using brittle materials. It also is a critical line of defense for protecting the occupants of the building.

The placement of the building on the site can have a major impact on its vulnerability. Ideally, the building is placed as far from the property lines as possible. This applies not only to the sides that are adjacent to streets, but the sides that are adjacent to adjoining properties, since it is not certain who will occupy the neighboring properties during the life of the building. A common, but unfortunate practice is to create a large plaza area in front of the building, but to leave little setback on the sides and rear of the building. Though this practice may increase the monumental character of the building, it also increases the vulnerability of the other three sides.

The shape of the building can have a contributing effect on the overall damage to the structure (see Figure 6-3). Re-entrant corners and overhangs are likely to trap the shock wave and amplify the effect of the air blast. Note that large or gradual re-entrant corners have less effect than small or sharp re-entrant corners and overhangs. The reflected pressure on the surface of a circular building is less intense than on a flat building. When curved surfaces are used, convex shapes are preferred over concave shapes. Terraces that are treated as roof systems subject to downward loads require careful framing and detailing to limit internal damage to supporting beams.

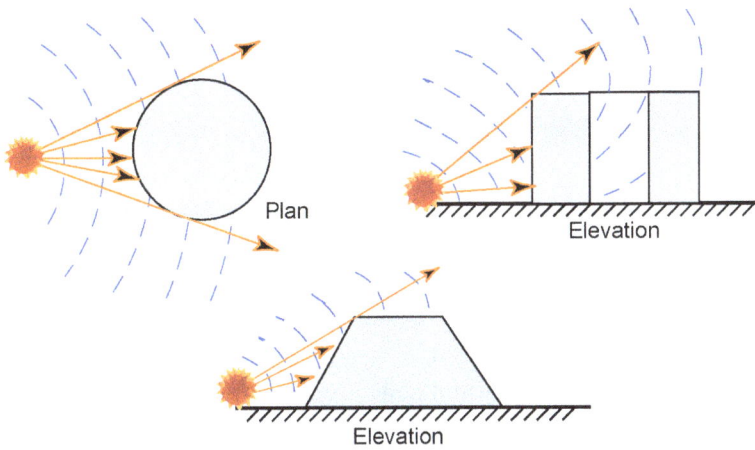

SHAPES THAT DISSIPATE AIR BLAST

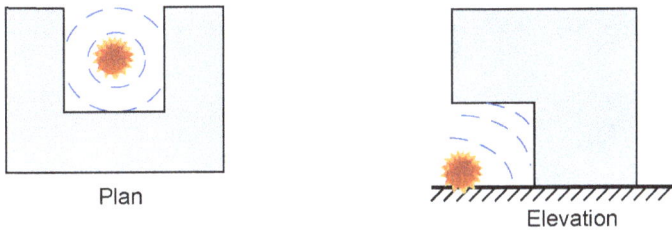

SHAPES THAT ACCENTUATE AIR BLAST

Figure 6-3   Schematics showing the effect of building shape on air-blast impacts

Generally, simple geometries and minimal ornamentation (which may become flying debris during an explosion) are recommended unless advanced structural analysis techniques are used. If ornamentation is used, it is preferable to use lightweight materials such as timber or plastic, which are less likely than brick, stone, or metal to become lethal projectiles in the event of an explosion.

Soil can be highly effective in reducing the impact of a major explosive attack. Bermed walls and buried roof tops have been found to be highly effective for military applications and can be effectively extended to conventional construction. This type of solution can also be effective in improving the energy efficiency of the building. Note that if this approach is taken, no parking can be permitted over the building.

Interior courtyards or atriums are other concepts for bringing light and a natural setting to the building without adding vulnerable openings to the exterior.

6.2.2   Building Interior

In terms of functional layout, unsecured areas such as the lobby, loading dock, mail room, garage, and retail areas need to be separated from the secured areas of the building . Ideally, these unsecured areas are placed exterior to the main building or along the edges of the building. For example, a separate lobby pavilion or loading dock area outside of the main footprint of the building (see Figure 6-4) provides enhanced protection against damage and potential building collapse in the event of an explosion at these locations. Similarly, placing parking areas outside the main footprint of the building can be highly effective in reducing the vulnerability to catastrophic collapse. If it is not possible to place

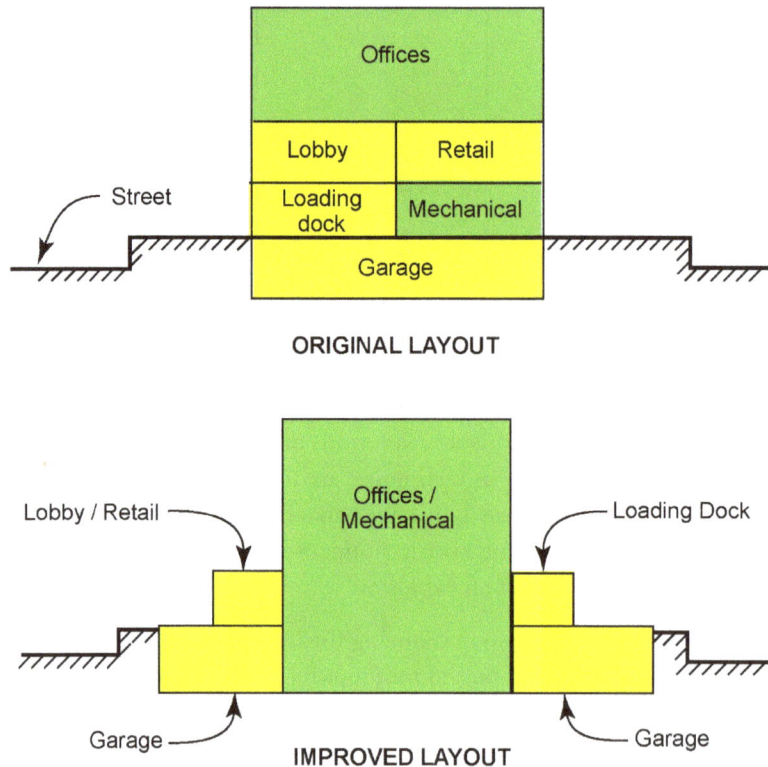

Figure 6-4   Schematics showing an example approach for improving the layout of adjacent unsecured and secured areas

vulnerable areas outside the main building footprint, they should be placed along the building exterior, and the building layout should be used to create internal "hard lines" or buffer zones. Secondary stairwells, elevator shafts, corridors, and storage areas should be located between public and secured areas.

When determining whether secured and unsecured areas are adjacent to one another, consider the layout on each floor and the relationship between floors. Secured occupied or critical areas should not be placed above or below unsecured areas.

Adequate queuing areas should be provided in front of lobby inspection stations so that visitors are not forced to stand outside during bad weather conditions or in a congested line inside a small lobby while waiting to enter the secured areas. Occupied areas or emergency functions should not be placed immediately adjacent to the lobby, but should be separated by a buffer area such as a storage area or corridor. The interior wall area and exposed structural columns in unsecured lobby areas should be minimized.

Vehicular queuing and inspection stations need to be accounted for in design of the loading docks and vehicle access points. These should be located outside the building along the curb or further away. A parking lane may be used for this purpose.

Emergency functions and elevator shafts are to be placed away from internal parking areas, loading docks and other high-risk areas. In the 1993 World Trade Center bombing incident, elevator shafts became chimneys, transmitting smoke and heat from the explosion in the basement to all levels of the building. This hindered evacuation and resulted in smoke inhalation injuries.

False ceilings, light fixtures, Venetian blinds, ductwork, air conditioners, and other nonstructural components may become flying debris in the event of an explosion. Wherever possible it is recommended that the design be simplified to limit these hazards. Placing heavy equipment such as air conditioners near the floor rather than the ceiling is one idea for limiting this hazard. Using fabric curtains or plastic vertical blinds rather than metal Venetian blinds, and using exposed ductwork as an architectural device are other ideas. Mechanically attaching light fixtures to the slab above as is done in high seismic areas is recommended.

Finally, the placement of furniture can have an effect on injury levels. Desks, conference tables, and other similar furniture should be placed as far from exterior windows facing streets as practical. Desks with computer monitors should be oriented away from the window to prevent injury due to the impact of the monitor.

6.2.3   Checklist – Architectural

✔ Use simple geometries without sharp re-entrant corners.

✔ Use lightweight nonstructural elements to reduce flying debris hazards.

✔ Place the building on the site as far from the perimeter as practical.

✔ Place unsecured areas exterior to the main structure or along the exterior of the building.

✔ Separate unsecured and secured areas horizontally and vertically using buffer zones and/or hardening of walls and floors.

✔ Provide sufficient queuing areas at lobby and delivery entrances.

✔ Limit nonstructural elements such as false ceilings and metal blinds on the interior.

✔ Mechanically fasten light fixtures to the floor system above.

✔ Place desks and conference tables as far from exterior windows as practical.

✔ Orient desks with computer monitors to face away from windows so the chair back faces the window, not the monitor.

6.2.4   Further Reading

The American Institute of Architects, 2001, *Building Security through Design: A Primer for Architects, Design Professionals, and their Clients*, The American Institute of Architects, Washington, D.C. http://www.aia.org/security

GSA, 1999, *Balancing Security and Openness: A Thematic Summary of a Symposium on Security and the Design of Public Buildings*, General Services Administration, Washington, D.C. http://hydra.gsa.gov/pbs/pc/gd_files/SecurityOpenness.pdf

Hart, S., 2002, In the Aftermath of September 11, the Urban Landscape Appears Vulnerable and Random: Architects and Consultants Focus on Risk Assessment and Security Through Design, *Architectural Record*, March 2002, pages 135-160, New York, New York. http://archrecord.construction.com/CONTEDUC/ARTICLES/03_02_1.asp

Nadel, B. A., 1998, Designing for Security, *Architectural Record*, March 1998, pages 145-148, 196-197, New York, New York. http:// www.archrecord.com/CONTEDUC/ARTICLES/3_98_1.asp

Council on Tall Buildings an Urban Habitat, 2002, *Building Safety Enhancement Guidebook*, Lehigh University, Bethlehem, Pennsylvania. http://www.ctbuh.org/

6.3   STRUCTURAL

Given the evolving nature of the terrorist threat, it is impossible to predict what threats may be of concern during the lifetime of the building; it is therefore prudent to provide protection against progressive collapse initiated by a localized structural failure caused by an undefined threat. Because of the catastrophic consequences of progressive collapse, incorporating these measures into the overall building design should be given the highest priority when considering structural design approaches for mitigating the effects of attacks.

Explicit design of secondary structural components to mitigate the direct effects of air-blast enhances life safety by providing protection against localized failure, flying debris, and air blast entering the building. It may also facilitate evacuation and rescue by limiting the overall damage level and improving access by emergency personnel.

Specific issues related to structural protection measures are discussed separately in the sections below.

6.3.1   Progressive Collapse

ASCE-7 defines three ways to approach the structural design of buildings to mitigate damage due to progressive collapse. Each is described below with an emphasis on how the method is applied in the situation where explosive loads are the initiating cause of collapse.

1. *Indirect Method*: Consider incorporating general structural integrity measures throughout the process of structural system selection, layout of walls and columns, member proportioning, and detailing of connections to enhance overall structural robustness. In lieu of calculations demonstrating the effects of explosions on buildings, one may use an implicit design approach that incorporates measures to increase the overall robustness of the structure. These measures are discussed in the sub-sections below on structural systems, structural layout, and structural elements. This minimum standard is likely to be the primary method used for design of the type of buildings that are the focus of this primer.

2. *Alternate-Load-Path Method*: Localize response by designing the structure to carry loads by means of an alternate load path in the event of the loss of a primary load-bearing component. The alternate-load-path method has been selected by agencies including the General Services Administration (GSA) as the preferred approach for preventing progressive collapse. This method provides a formal check of the capability of the structure to resist collapse following the removal of specific elements, such as a building column at the building perimeter. The method does not require characterization of the explosive threat. The structural engineer can usually perform the necessary analyses, with or without guidance from a protective design consultant. However, the analysis is likely to benefit from advice of the protective design consultant regarding element loss scenarios that should be considered in design.

3. *Specific Local-Resistance Method*: Explicitly design critical vertical load-bearing building components to resist the design-level explosive forces. Explosive loads for a defined threat may be explicitly considered in design by using nonlinear dynamic analysis methods. These are discussed below in the subsection on direct design methods with additional information in the subsection on structural elements. Blast-mitigating structural design or hardening generally focuses on the structural members on the lower floor levels that are closest to defined stationary exterior vehicle weapon threats.

Useful references are provided at the end of this section that directly relate to progressive collapse prevention.

6.3.2   Building Structural Systems

In the selection of the structural system, consider both the direct effects of air-blast and the potential for progressive collapse in the event that a critical structural component fails.

The characteristics of air-blast loading have been previously discussed. To resist the direct effects of air-blast, the structural characteristics listed below are desirable.

○ **Mass**. Lightweight construction is unsuitable for providing air-blast resistance. For example, a building with steel deck (without concrete fill) roof construction will have little air-blast resistance.

○ **Shear Capacity.** Primary members and/or their connections should ensure that flexural capacity is achieved prior to shear failure. Avoiding brittle shear failure significantly increases the structure's ability to absorb energy.

○ **Capacity for Reversing Loads.** Primary members and their connections should resist upward pressure. Certain systems such as pre-stressed concrete may have little resistance to upward forces. Seated connection systems for steel and precast concrete may also have little resistance to uplift. The use of headed studs is recommended for affixing concrete fill over steel deck to beams for uplift resistance.

To reduce the risk of progressive collapse in the event of the loss of structural elements, the structural traits listed below should be incorporated.

○ **Redundancy.** The incorporation of redundant load paths in the vertical-load-carrying system helps to ensure that alternate load paths are available in the event of failure of structural elements.

○ **Ties.** An integrated system of ties in perpendicular directions along the principal lines of structural framing can serve to redistribute loads during catastrophic events.

○ **Ductility.** In a catastrophic event, members and their connections may have to maintain their strength while undergoing large deformations.

Historically, the preferred material for explosion-mitigating construction is cast-in-place reinforced concrete. This is the material used for military bunkers, and the military has performed extensive research and testing of its performance. Reinforced concrete has a number of attributes that make it the construction material of choice. It has significant mass, which improves response to explosions, because the mass is often mobilized only after the pressure wave is significantly diminished, reducing deformations. Members can be readily proportioned and reinforced for ductile behavior. The construction is unparalleled in its ability to achieve continuity between the members. Finally, concrete columns are less susceptible to global buckling in the event of the loss of a floor system.

Current testing programs are investigating the effectiveness of various conventional building systems; however, in general the level of protection that may be a achieved using these materials is lower than what is achieved using well-designed, cast-in-place, reinforced concrete. The performance of a conventional steel frame with concrete fill over metal deck depends on the connection details. Pre-tensioned or post-tensioned construction provides little capacity for abnormal loading patterns and load reversals. The resistance of load-bearing wall structures varies to a great extent. More information about the response of these systems is described in the subsection on structural elements and in the section on exterior cladding in Section 6.4, Exterior Envelope.

6.3.3 Structural Layout

To enhance the overall robustness of the structure, the measures listed below are recommended.

○ In frame structures, column spacing should be limited. Large column spacing decreases likelihood that the structure will be able to redistribute load in event of column failure.

○ The exterior bay is the most vulnerable to damage, particularly for buildings that are close to public streets. It is also less capable of redistributing loads in the event of member loss, since two-way load distribution is not possible. It is desirable to have a shallow bay adjacent to the building exterior to limit the extent of damage.

○ Use of transfer girders is strongly discouraged. Loss of a transfer girder or one of its supports can destabilize a significant area of the building. Transfer girders are often found at the building exterior to accommodate loading docks or generous entries, increasing their vulnerability to air-blast effects. It is highly desirable to add redundant transfer systems where transfer girders are required.

○ In bearing-wall systems that rely primarily on interior cross-walls, interior longitudinal walls should be periodically spaced to enhance stability and to control the lateral progression of damage.

○ In bearing-wall systems that rely on exterior walls, perpendicular walls or substantial pilasters should be provided at a regular spacing to control the amount of wall that is likely to be affected.

6.3.4 Direct Design Methods

The direct design approach (Figure 6-5) to be used for the structural protective measures is to first design the building for conventional loads, then evaluate the structure's response to explosive loads and augment the design, if needed. Finally, the designer must make sure that all conventional load requirements are still met. This approach ensures that the design meets all the requirements for gravity and natural hazards in addition to air-blast effects. Take note that measures taken to mitigate explosive loads may reduce the structure's performance under other types of loads, and therefore an iterative approach may be needed. As an example, increased mass generally increases the design forces for seismic loads, whereas increased mass generally improves performance under explosive loads. Careful consideration between the

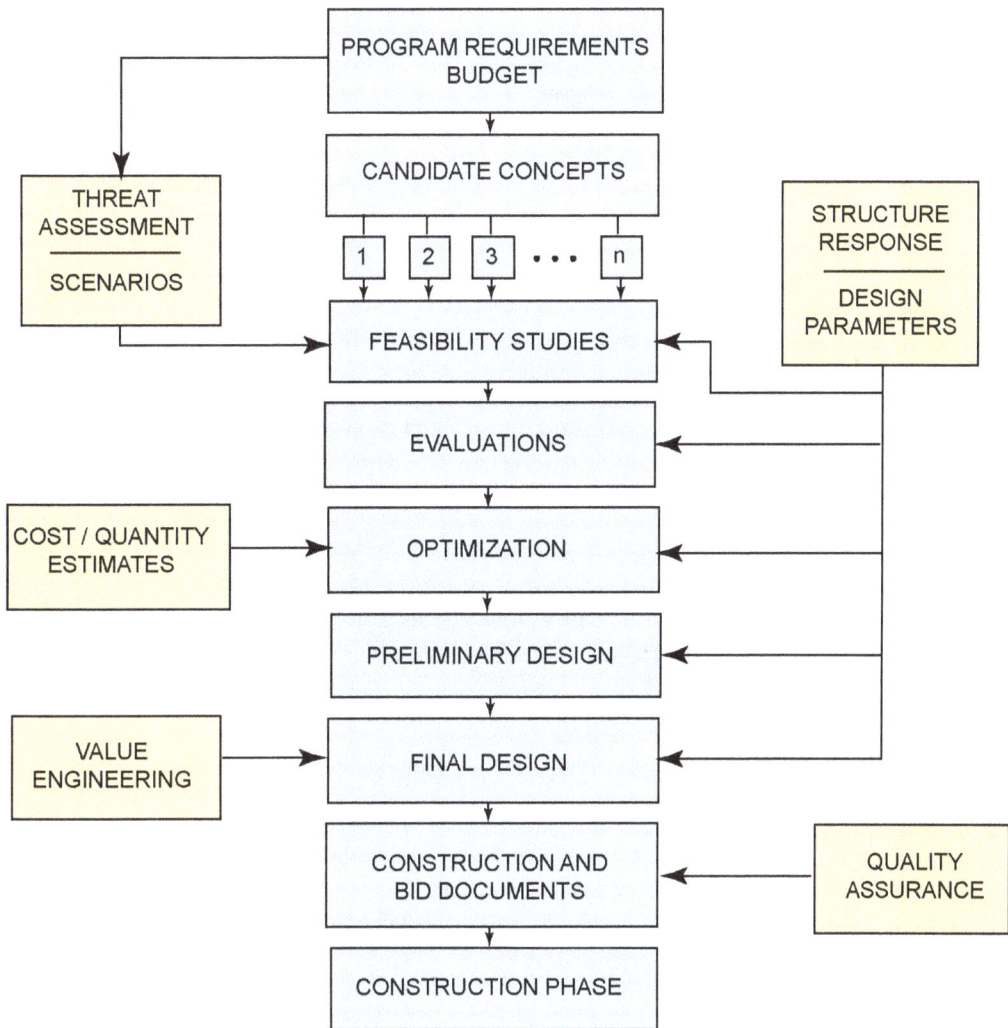

Figure 6-5   Direct design process flow chart

protective design consultant and the structural engineer is needed to provide an optimized design.

Nonlinear dynamic analysis techniques are similar to those currently used in advanced seismic analysis. Analytical models range from hand-book methods to equivalent single-degree-of-freedom (SDOF) models to finite element (FE) representation. For SDOF and FE methods, numerical computation requires adequate resolution in space and time to account for the high-intensity, short-duration loading and nonlinear response (Figure 6-6). Difficulties involve the selection of the model

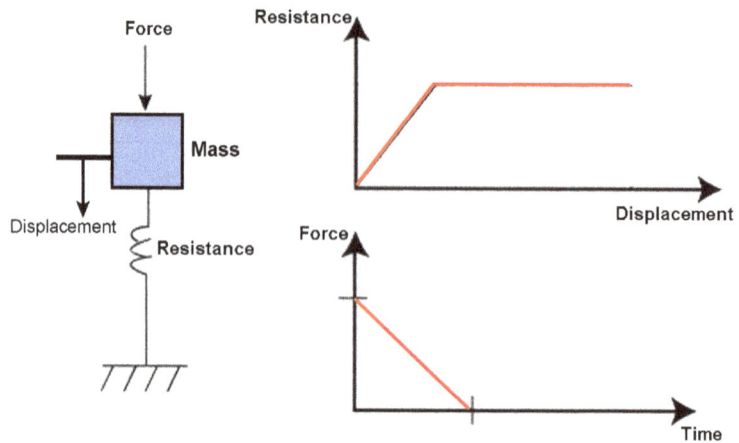

Figure 6-6   Single-degree-of-feedom model for explosive loads. Note variation of force and displacement with time.

and appropriate failure modes, and finally, the interpretation of the results for structural design details. Whenever possible, results are checked against data from tests and experiments for similar structures and loadings.

Charts are available that provide damage estimates for various types of construction, as a function of peak pressure and peak impulse, based on analysis or empirical data. Military design handbooks typically provide this type of design information.

Components such as beams, slabs, or walls can often be modeled by a SDOF system and the governing equation of motion solved by using numerical methods. There are also charts available in text books and military handbooks for linearly decaying loads, which provide the peak response and circumvent the need to solve differential equations. These charts require only knowledge of the fundamental period of the element, its ultimate resistance force, the peak pressure applied to the element, and the equivalent linear decay time to evaluate the peak displacement response of the system. The design of the anchorage and supporting structural system can be evaluated by using the ultimate flexural capacity obtained from the dynamic analysis.

For SDOF systems, material behavior can be modeled using idealized elastic, perfectly-plastic stress-deformation functions, based on actual structural support conditions and strain-rate-enhanced material properties. The model properties selected provide the same peak displacement and fundamental period as the actual structural system in flexure. Furthermore, the mass and the resistance functions are multiplied by mass and load factors, which estimate the actual portion of the mass or load participating in the deflection of the member along its span.

For more complex elements, the engineer must resort to finite-element numerical time integration techniques and/or explosive testing. The time and cost of the analysis cannot be ignored when choosing design procedures. Because the design process is a sequence of iterations, the cost of analysis must be justified in terms of benefits to the project and increased confidence in the reliability of the results. In some cases, an SDOF approach will be used for the preliminary design, and a more sophisticated approach using finite elements, and/or explosive testing may be used for the final verification of the design.

A dynamic nonlinear approach is more likely than a static approach to provide a section that meets the design constraints of the project. Elastic static calculations are likely to give overly conservative design solutions if the peak pressure is considered without the effect of load duration. By using dynamic calculations instead of static, we are able to account for the very short duration of the loading. Because the peak pressure levels are so high, it is important to account for the short duration to properly model the structural response. In addition, the inertial effect included in dynamic computations greatly improves response. This is because by the time the mass is mobilized, the loading is greatly diminished, enhancing response. Furthermore, by accepting that damage occurs it is possible to account for the energy absorbed by ductile systems through plastic deformation. Finally, because the loading is so rapid, it is possible to enhance the material strength to account for strain-rate effects.

In dynamic nonlinear analysis, response is evaluated by comparing the ductility (i.e., the peak displacement divided by the elastic limit displacement) and/or support rotation (the angle between the support and the point of peak deflection) to empirically established maximum values that have been established by the military through explosive testing. Note that these values are typically based on limited testing and are not well defined within the industry at this time. Maximum permissible values vary, depending on the material and the acceptable damage level.

Levels of damage computed by means of analysis may be described by the terms minor, moderate, or major, depending on the peak ductility, support rotation and collateral effects. A brief description of each damage level is given below.

> *Minor:* Nonstructural failure of building elements such as windows, doors, cladding, and false ceilings. Injuries may be expected, and fatalities are possible but unlikely.

> *Moderate:* Structural damage is confined to a localized area and is usually repairable. Structural failure is limited to secondary structural members such as beams, slabs, and non-load-bearing walls. However, if the building has been designed for loss of primary members, localized loss of columns may be accommodated. Injuries and possible fatalities are expected.

> *Major:* Loss of primary structural components such as columns or transfer girders precipitates loss of additional adjacent members that are adjacent to or above the lost member. In this case, extensive fatalities are expected. Building is usually not repairable.

Generally, moderate damage at the design threat level is a reasonable design goal for new construction.

6.3.5   Structural Elements

Because direct explosion effects decay rapidly with distance, the local response of structural components is the dominant concern. General principles governing the design of critical components are discussed below.

6.3.5.1   Exterior Frame

There are two primary considerations for the exterior frame. The first is to design the exterior columns to resist the direct effects of the specified threats. The second is to ensure that the exterior frame has sufficient structural integrity to accept localized failure without initiating progressive collapse. The former is discussed in this section, the latter in the sub-section on structural integrity. Exterior cladding and glazing issues are discussed in Section 6.4, Building Envelope.

Because columns do not have much surface area, air-blast loads on columns tend to be mitigated by "clear-time effects". This refers to the pressure wave washing around these slender tall members, and consequently the entire duration of the pressure wave does not act upon them. On the other hand, the critical threat is directly across from them, so they are loaded with the peak reflected pressure, which is typically several times larger than the incident or overpressure wave that is propagating through the air.

For columns subjected to a vehicle weapon threat on an adjacent street, buckling and shear are the primary effects to be considered in analysis. If a very large weapon is detonated close to a column, shattering of the concrete due to multiple tensile reflections within the concrete section can destroy its integrity.

Buckling is a concern if lateral support is lost due to the failure of a supporting floor system. This is particularly important for buildings that are close to public streets. In this case, exterior columns should be capable of spanning two or more stories without buckling. Slender steel columns are at substantially greater risk than are concrete columns.

Confinement of concrete using columns with closely spaced closed ties or spiral reinforcing will improve shear capacity, improve the performance of lap splices in the event of loss of concrete cover, and greatly enhance column ductility. The potential benefit from providing closely spaced closed ties in exterior concrete columns is very high relative to the cost of the added reinforcement.

For steel columns, splices should be placed as far above grade level as practical. It is recommended that splices at exterior columns that are not specifically designed to resist air-blast loads employ complete-penetration welded flanges. Welding details, materials, and procedures should be selected to ensure toughness.

For a package weapon, column breach is a major consideration. Some suggestions for mitigating this concern are listed below.

- Do not use exposed columns that are fully or partially accessible from the building exterior. Arcade columns should be avoided.
- Use an architectural covering that is at least six inches from the structural member. This will make it considerably more difficult to place a weapon directly against the structure. Because explosive pressures decay so rapidly, every inch of distance will help to protect the column.

Load- bearing reinforced concrete wall construction can provide a considerable level of protection if adequate reinforcement is provided to achieve ductile behavior. This may be an appropriate solution for the parts of the building that are closest to the secured perimeter line (within twenty feet). Masonry is a much more brittle material that is capable of generating highly hazardous flying debris in the event of an explosion. Its use is generally discouraged for new construction.

Spandrel beams of limited depth generally do well when subjected to air blast. In general, edge beams are very strongly encouraged at the perimeter of concrete slab construction to afford frame action for redistribution of vertical loads and to enhance the shear connection of floors to columns.

6.3.5.2   Roof System

The primary loading on the roof is the downward air-blast pressure. The exterior bay roof system on the side(s) facing an exterior threat is the most critical. The air-blast pressure on the interior bays is less intense, so the roof there may require less hardening. Secondary loads include upward pressure due to the air blast penetrating through openings and upward suction during the negative loading phase. The upward pressure may have an increased duration due to multiple reflections of the internal air-blast wave. It is conservative to consider the downward and upward loads separately.

The preferred system is cast-in-place reinforced concrete with beams in two directions. If this system is used, beams should have continuous top and bottom reinforcement with tension lap splices. Stirrups to develop the bending capacity of the beams closely spaced along the entire span are recommended.

Somewhat lower levels of protection are afforded by conventional steel beam construction with a steel deck and concrete fill slab. The performance of this system can be enhanced by use of normal-weight concrete fill instead of lightweight fill, increasing the gauge of welded wire fabric reinforcement, and making the connection between the slab and beams with shear connector studs. Since it is anticipated that the slab capacity will exceed that of the supporting beams, beam end connections should be capable of developing the ultimate flexural capacity of the beams to avoid brittle failure. Beam-to-column connections should be capable of resisting upward as well as downward forces.

Precast and pre-/post-tensioned systems are generally considered less desirable, unless members and connections are capable of resisting upward forces generated by rebound from the direct pressure and/or the suction from the negative pressure phase of the air blast.

Concrete flat slab/plate systems are also less desirable because of the potential of shear failure at the columns. When flat slab/plate systems are used, they should include features to enhance their punching shear resistance. Continuous bottom reinforcement should be provided through columns in two directions to retain the slab in the event that punching shear failure occurs. Edge beams should be provided at the building exterior.

Lightweight systems, such as untopped steel deck or wood frame construction, are considered to afford minimal resistance to air-blast. These systems are prone to failure due to their low capacity for downward and uplift pressures.

6.3.5.3   Floor System

The floor system design should consider three possible scenarios: air-blast loading, redistributing load in the event of loss of a column or wall support below, and the ability to arrest debris falling from the floor or roof above.

For structures in which the interior is secured against bombs of moderate size by package inspection, the primary concern is the exterior bay framing. For buildings that are separated from a public street only by a sidewalk, the uplift pressures from a vehicle weapon may be significant enough to cause possible failure of the exterior bay floors for several levels above ground. Special concern exists in the case of vertical irregularities in the architectural system, either where the exterior wall is set back from the floor above or where the structure steps back to form terraces. The recommendations of Section 6.3.5.2 for roof systems apply to these areas.

Structural hardening of floor systems above unsecured areas of the building such as lobbies, loading docks, garages, mailrooms, and retail spaces should be considered. In general, critical or heavily occupied areas should not be placed underneath unsecured areas, since it is virtually impossible to prevent against localized breach in conventional construction for package weapons placed on the floor.

Precast panels are problematic because of their tendency to fail at the connections. Pre-/post-tensioned systems tend to fail in a brittle manner if stressed much beyond their elastic limit. These systems are also not able to accept upward loads without additional reinforcement. If pre-/post-tensioned systems are used, continuous mild steel needs to be added to the top and the bottom faces to provide the ductility needed to resist explosion loads.

Flat slab/plate systems are also less desirable because of limited two way action and the potential for shear failure at the columns. When flat slab/plate systems are employed, they should include features to enhance their punching shear resistance, and continuous bottom reinforcement should be provided across columns to resist progressive collapse. Edge beams should be provided at the building exterior.

6.3.5.4   Interior Columns

Interior columns in unsecured areas are subject to many of the same issues as exterior columns. If possible, columns should not be accessible within these areas. If they are accessible, then obscure their location or impose a standoff to the structural component through the use of cladding. Methods of hardening columns (already discussed under Section 6.3.5.1, Exterior Frame) include using closely spaced ties, spiral reinforcement, and architectural covering at least six inches from the structural elements. Composite steel and concrete sections or steel plating of concrete columns can provide higher levels of protection. Columns in unsecured areas should be designed to span two or three stories without buckling in the event that the floor below and possibly above the detonation area have failed, as previously discussed.

6.3.5.5   Interior Walls

Interior walls surrounding unsecured spaces are designed to contain the explosive effects within the unsecured areas. Ideally, unsecured areas are located adjacent to the building exterior so that the explosive pressure may be vented outward as well.

Fully grouted CMU (concrete masonry unit) block walls that are well reinforced vertically and horizontally and adequately supported laterally are a common solution. Anchorage at the top and bottom of walls should be capable of developing the full flexural capacity of the wall. Lateral support at the top of the walls may be achieved using steel angles anchored into the floor system above. Care should be taken to terminate bars at the top of the wall with hooks or heads and to ensure that the upper course of block is filled solid with grout. The base of the wall may be anchored by reinforcing bar dowels.

Interior walls can also be effective in resisting progressive collapse if they are designed properly with sufficient load-bearing capacity and are tied into the floor systems below and above.

This design for hardened interior wall construction is also recommended for primary egress routes to protect against explosions, fire, and other hazards trapping occupants.

6.3.6   Checklist – Structural

✔ Incorporate measures to prevent progressive collapse.

✔ Design floor systems for uplift in unsecured areas and in exterior bays that may pose a hazard to occupants.

✔ Limit column spacing.

✔ Avoid transfer girders.

✔ Use two-way floor and roof systems.

✔ Use fully grouted, heavily reinforced CMU block walls that are properly anchored in order to separate unsecured areas from critical functions and occupied secured areas.

✔ Use dynamic nonlinear analysis methods for design of critical structural components.

6.3.7 Further Reading

Listed below are publicly available references on structural hardening. Other references are given in the chapter on Weapons Effects. Existing design criteria are given in the chapter on Design Approach.

Mays, G.C. and Smith, P.D. (editors), 1995, *Blast Effects on Buildings: Design of Buildings to Optimize Resistance to Blast Loading.*, American Society of Civil Engineers, Reston, Virginia.

Conrath, E., et al., 1999, *Structural Design for Physical Security: State of the Practice.* Structural Engineering Institute of American Society of Civil Engineers, Reston, Virginia.

Ettouney, M., Smilowitz, R., and Rittenhouse, T., 1996, Blast Resistant Design of Commercial Buildings. *Practice Periodical on Structural Design and Construction*, Vol. 1, No. 1, American Society of Civil Engineers. http://ojps.aip.org/dbt/dbt.jsp?KEY=PPSCFX&Volume=1&Issue=1 A preprint of the final article is available at http://www.wai.com/AppliedScience/Blast/blast-struct-design.html

American Society of Civil Engineers,1997, *Design of Blast Resistant Buildings in Petrochemical Facilities.* American Society of Civil Engineers, Reston, Virginia.

American Society of Civil Engineers, 2002, *Vulnerability and Protection of Infrastructure Systems: The State of the Art.* An ASCE Journals Special Publication compiling articles from 2002 and earlier available online https://ascestore.aip.org/OA_HTML/aipCCtpSctDspRte.jsp?section=10123

References on Progressive Collapse:

American Society of Civil Engineers, 2002, *Minimum Design Loads for Buildings and Other Structures*, ASCE-7, Reston Virginia, ISBN: 0-7844-0624-3, http://www.asce.org/publications/dsp_pubdetails.cfm?puburl=http://www.pubs.asce.org/ASCE7.html?9991330

General Services Administration, 2000, *Progressive Collapse Analysis and Design Guidelines for New Federal Office Buildings and Major Modernization Projects*, U.S. General Services Administration, Washington, D.C. http://www.oca.gsa.gov/about_progressive_collapse/progcollapse.php

Burnett, E. F. P., 1975, *The Avoidance of Progressive Collapse, Regulatory Approaches to the Problem*, National Bureau of Standards, Washington D.C.

Conrath, E., 2000, *Interim Antiterrorism/Force Protection Construction Standards – Progressive Collapse Guidance*, Contact US Army Corps of Engineers Protective Design Center, ATTN: CENWO-ED-ST, 215 N. 17th Street, Omaha, Nebraska, 68102-4978, phone: (402) 221-4918.

6.4 BUILDING ENVELOPE

Exterior wall/cladding and window systems and other openings are discussed in this section. For a discussion of the roof and exterior frame, see Section 6.3.5, Structural Elements.

6.4.1 Exterior Wall/Cladding Design

The exterior walls provide the first line of defense against the intrusion of the air-blast pressure and hazardous debris into the building. They are subject to direct reflected pressures from an explosive threat located directly across from the wall along the secured perimeter line. If the building is more than four stories high, it may be advantageous to consider the reduction in pressure with height due to the increased distance and angle of incidence. The objective of design at a minimum is to ensure that these members fail in a ductile mode such as flexure rather than a brittle mode such as shear. The walls also need to be able to resist the loads transmitted by the windows and doors. It is not uncommon, for instance, for bullet-resistant windows to have a higher ultimate capacity than the walls to which they are attached. Beyond ensuring a ductile failure mode, the exterior wall may be designed to resist the actual or reduced pressure levels of the defined threat. Note that special reinforcing and anchors should be provided around blast-resistant window and door frames.

Poured-in-place, reinforced concrete will provide the highest level of protection, but solutions like pre-cast concrete, CMU block, and metal stud systems may also be used to achieve lower levels of protection.

For pre-cast panels, consider a minimum thickness of five inches exclusive of reveals, with two-way, closely spaced reinforcing bars to increase ductility and reduce the chance of flying concrete fragments. The objective is to reduce the loads transmitted into the connections, which need to be designed to resist the ultimate flexural resistance of the panels. Also, connections into the structure should provide as straight a line of load transmittal as practical.

For CMU block walls, use eight-inch block walls, fully grouted with vertically centered heavy reinforcing bars and horizontal reinforcement placed at each layer. Connections into the structure should be designed to resist the ultimate lateral capacity of the wall. For infill walls, avoid transferring loads into the columns if they are primary load-carrying elements. The connection details may be very difficult to construct. It will be difficult to have all the blocks fit over the bars near the top, and it will be difficult to provide the required lateral restraint at the top connection. A preferred system is to have a continuous exterior CMU wall that laterally bears against the floor system. For increased protection, consider using 12-inch blocks with two layers of vertical reinforcement.

For metal stud systems, use metal studs back-to-back and mechanically attached, to minimize lateral torsional effects. To catch exterior cladding fragments, attach a wire mesh or steel sheet to the exterior side of the metal stud system. The supports of the wall should be designed to resist the ultimate lateral out-of-plane bending capacity load of the system.

Brick veneers and other nonstructural elements attached to the building exterior are to be avoided or have strengthened connections to limit flying debris and to improve emergency egress by ensuring that exits remain passable.

6.4.2 Window Design

Windows, once the sole responsibility of the architect, become a structural issue when explosive effects are taken into consideration. In designing windows to mitigate the effects of explosions they should first be designed to resist conventional loads and then be checked for explosive load effects and balanced design.

Balanced or capacity design philosophy means that the glass is designed to be no stronger than the weakest part of the overall window system, failing at pressure levels that do not exceed those of the frame, anchorage, and supporting wall system. If the glass is stronger than the supporting members, then the window is likely to fail with the whole panel entering into the building as a single unit, possibly with the frame, anchorage, and the wall attached. This failure mode is considered more hazardous than if the glass fragments enter the building, provided that the fragments are designed to minimize injuries. By using a damage-limiting approach, the damage sequence and extent of damage can be controlled.

Windows are typically the most vulnerable portion of any building. Though it may be impractical to design all the windows to resist a large-scale explosive attack, it is desirable to limit the amount of hazardous glass breakage to reduce the injuries. Typical annealed glass windows break at low pressure and impulse levels and the shards created by broken windows are responsible for many of the injuries incurred during a large-scale explosive attack.

Designing windows to provide protection against the effects of explosions can be effective in reducing the glass laceration injuries in areas that are not directly across from the weapon. For a large-scale vehicle weapon, this pressure range is expected on the sides of surrounding buildings not facing the explosion or for smaller explosions in which pressures drop more rapidly with distance. Generally, it is not known on which side of the building the attack will occur, so all sides need to be protected. Window protection should be evaluated on a case-by-case basis by a qualified protective design consultant to develop a solution that meets established objectives. Several recommended solutions for the design of the window systems to reduce injuries to building occupants are provided in Figure 6-7.

Several approaches that can be taken to limit glass laceration injuries. One way is to reduce the number and size of windows. If blast-resistant walls are used, then fewer and/or smaller windows will allow less air blast to enter the building, thus reducing the interior damage and injuries. Specific examples of how to incorporate these ideas into the design of a new building include (1) limiting the number of windows on the lower floors where the pressures would be higher during an external explosion; (2) using an internal atrium design with windows facing

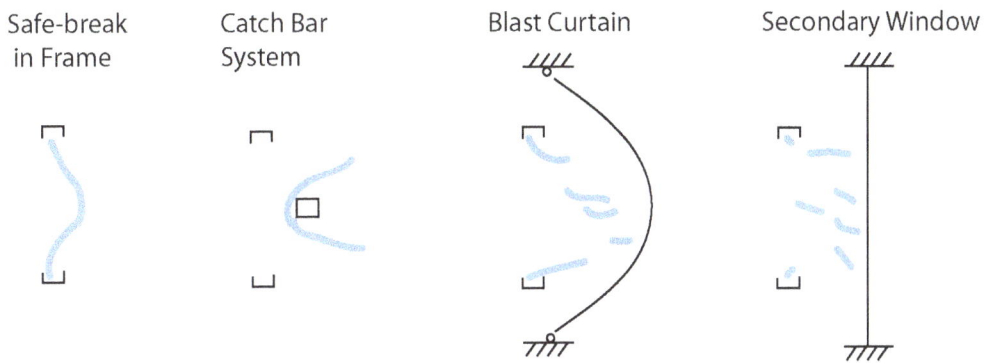

Safe-break in Frame	Catch Bar System	Blast Curtain	Secondary Window

Figure 6-7   Safe laminated-glass systems and failure modes

inward, not outward; (3) using clerestory windows, which are close to the ceiling, above the heads of the occupants; and (4) angling the windows away from the curb to reduce the pressure levels.

Glass curtain-wall, butt glazed, and Pilkington type systems have been found to perform surprisingly well in recent explosive tests with low explosive loads. In particular, glass curtain wall systems have been shown to accept larger deformations without the glass breaking hazardously, compared to rigidly supported punched window systems. Some design modifications to the connections, details, and member sizes may be required to optimize the performance.

6.4.2.1   Glass Design

Glass is often the weakest part of a building, breaking at low pressures compared to other components such as the floors, walls, or columns. Past incidents have shown that glass breakage and associated injuries may extend many thousands of feet in large external explosions. High-velocity glass fragments have been shown to be a major contributor to injuries in such incidents. For incidents within downtown city areas, falling glass poses a major hazard to passersby and prolongs post-incident rescue and clean-up efforts by leaving tons of glass debris on the street. At this time, the issue of exterior debris is largely ignored by existing criteria.

As part of the damage-limiting approach, glass failure is not quantified in terms of whether breakage occurs or not, but rather by the hazard it causes to the occupants. Two failure modes that reduce the hazard posed by window glass are

○ glass that breaks but is retained by the frame and

○ glass fragments exit the frame and fall within three to ten feet of the window.

The glass performance conditions are defined based on empirical data from explosive tests performed in a cubical space with a 10- foot dimension (Table 6-1). The performance condition ranges from 1, which corresponds to not breaking, to 5, which corresponds to hazardous flying debris at a distance of 10 feet from the window (see Figure 6-8). Generally a performance condition 3 or 4 is considered acceptable for buildings that are not at high risk of attack. At this level, the window breaks and fragments fly into the building but land harmlessly within 10 feet of the window or impact a witness panel 10 feet away, no more than 2 feet above the floor level. The design goal is to achieve a performance level less than 4 for 90 percent of the windows.

Table 6-1: Performance Conditions for Windows

Performance Condition	Protection Level	Hazard Level	Description of Window Glazing
1	Safe	None	Glazing does not break. No visible damage to glazing or frame.
2	Very High	None	Glazing cracks but is retained by the frame. Dusting or very small fragments near sill or on floor acceptable.
3a	High	Very Low	Glass cracks. Fragments enter space and land on floor no further than 1 meter (3.3 feet) from window.
3b	High	Low	Glazing cracks. Fragments enter space and land on floor no further than 3 meters (10 feet) from the window.
4	Medium	Medium	Glazing cracks. Fragments enter space and land on floor and impact a vertical witness panel at a distance of no more than 3 m (10 feet) from the window at a height no greater than 2 feet above the floor.
5	Low	High	Glazing cracks and window system fails catastrophically. Fragments enter space impacting a vertical witness panel at a distance of no more than 3 meters (10 feet) from the window at a height greater than 0.6 meters (2 feet) above the floor.

The preferred solution for new construction is to use laminated annealed (i.e., float) glass with structural sealant around the inside perimeter. For insulated units, only the inner pane needs to be laminated. The lamination holds the shards of glass together in explosive

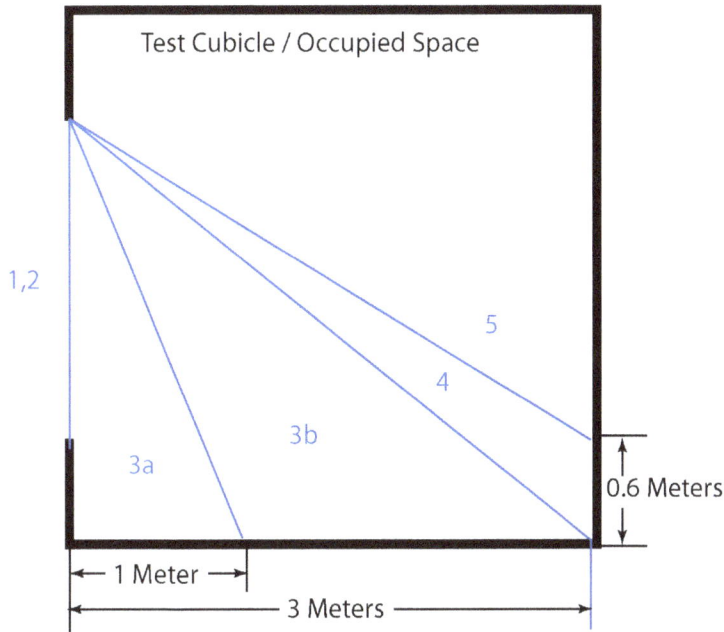

Figure 6-8   Plan view of test cubicle showing glass performance conditions as a function of distance from test window.

events, reducing its ability to cause laceration injuries. The structural sealant helps to hold the pane in the frame for higher loads. Annealed glass is used because it has a breaking strength that is about one-half that of heat-strengthened glass and about one-fourth as strong as tempered glass. Using annealed glass becomes particularly important for buildings with lightweight exterior walls using for instance, metal studs, dry wall, and brick façade. Use the thinnest overall glass thickness that is acceptable based on conventional load requirements. Also, it is important to use an interlayer thickness that is 60 mil thick rather than 30 mil thick, as is used in conventional applications. This layup has been shown to perform well in low-pressure regions (i.e., under about 5 psi). If a 60 mil polyvinyl butaryl (PVB) layer is used, the tension membrane forces into the framing members need to be considered in design.

To make sure that the components supporting the glass are stronger than the glass itself, specify a window breakage strength that is high compared to what is used in conventional design. The breakage strength in window design may be specified as a function of the number of windows expected to break at that load. For instance, in conventional design, it is typical to use a breakage pressure corresponding to eight breaks out of 1000. When a lot of glass breakage is expected, such as for an explosive incident, use a pressure corresponding to 750 breaks out of 1000 to increase confidence that the frame does not fail, too. Glass breakage strength values may be obtained from window manufacturers.

6.4.2.2   Mullion Design

The frame members connecting adjoining windows are referred to as mullions. These members may be designed in two ways. Using a static approach, the breaking strength of the window glass is applied to the mullion; alternatively, a dynamic load can be applied using the peak pressure and impulse values. The static approach may lead to a design that is not practical, because the mullion can become very deep and heavy, driving up the weight and cost of the window system. It may also not be consistent with the overall architectural objectives for the project.

As with frames, it is good engineering practice to limit the number of interlocking parts used for the mullion.

6.4.2.3   Frame and Anchorage Design

Window frames need to retain the glass so that the entire pane does not become a single large unit of flying debris. It also needs to be designed to resist the breaking stress of the window glass.

To retain the glass in the frame, a minimum of a ¼-inch bead of structural sealant (e.g., silicone) should be used around the inner perimeter of the window. The allowable tensile strength should be at least 20 psi. Also, the window bite (i.e., the depth of window captured by the frame) needs to be at least ½ inch. The structural sealant recommendations should be determined on a case-by-case basis. In some applications, the structural sealant may govern the overall design of the window system.

Frame and anchorage design is performed by applying the breaking strength of the window to the frame and the fasteners. In most conventionally designed buildings, the frames will be aluminum. In some applications, steel frames are used. Also, in lobby areas where large panes of glass are used, a larger bite with more structural sealant may be needed.

Inoperable windows are generally recommended for air-blast mitigating designs. However, some operable window designs are conceptually viable. For instance, designs in which the window rotates about a horizontal hinge at the head or sill and opens in the outward direction may perform adequately. In these designs, the window will slam shut in an explosion event. If this type of design is used, the governing design parameter may be the capacity of the hinges and/or hardware.

6.4.2.4 Wall Design

The supporting wall response should be checked using approaches similar to those for frames and mullions. It does not make sense, and is potentially highly hazardous, to have a wall system that is weaker than windows. Remember that the maximum strength of any wall system needs to be at least equal to the window strength. If the walls are unable to accept the loads transmitted by the mullions, the mullions may need to be anchored into the structural slabs or spandrel beams. Anchoring into columns is generally discouraged, because it increases the tributary area of lateral load that is transferred into the columns and may cause instability.

The balanced-design approach is particularly challenging in the design of ballistic-resistant and forced-entry-resistant windows, which consist of one or more inches of glass and polycarbonate. These windows can easily become stronger than the supporting wall. In these cases, the windows may need to be designed for the design threat air-blast pressure levels under the implicit assumption that balanced-design conditions will not be met for larger loads.

6.4.2.5 Multi-hazard Considerations

Under normal operating conditions, windows perform several functions listed below.

- They permit light to enter building.
- They save energy by reducing thermal transmission.
- They make the building quieter by reducing acoustic transmission.

Explosions are one of a number of abnormal loading conditions that the building may undergo. Some of the others are

- fire,
- earthquake,
- hurricane,
- gun fire, and
- forced entry.

When developing a protection strategy for windows to mitigate the effects of a particular explosion threat scenario, it is important to consider how this protection may interfere with some of these other functions or other explosion threat scenarios. Some questions that may be worthwhile to consider are listed below.

○ If an internal explosion occurs, will the upgraded windows increase smoke inhalation injuries by preventing the smoke to vent through windows that would normally break in an explosion event?

○ If a fire occurs, will it be more difficult to break the protected windows to vent the building and gain access to the injured?

○ Will a window upgrade that is intended to protect the occupants worsen the hazard to passersby?

6.4.3   Other Openings

Doors, louvers, and other openings in the exterior envelope should be designed so that the anchorage into the supporting structure has a lateral capacity greater than that of the element.

There are two general recommendations for doors.

○ Doors should open outward so that they bear against the jamb during the positive-pressure phase of the air-blast loading.

○ Door jambs can be filled with concrete to improve their resistance.

For louvers that provide air to sensitive equipment, some recommendations are given below.

○ Provide a baffle in front of the louver so that the air blast does not have direct line-of-sight access through the louver.

○ Provide a grid of steel bars properly anchored into the structure behind the louver to catch any debris generated by the louver or other flying fragments.

6.4.4   Checklist – Building Envelope

Cladding

✔ Use the thinnest panel thickness that is acceptable for conventional loads.

✔ Design cladding supports and the supporting structure to resist the ultimate lateral resistance of the panel.

✔ Design cladding connections to have as direct a load transmission path into the main structure as practical. A good transmission path minimizes shear and torsional response.

✔ Avoid framing cladding into columns and other primary vertical load-carrying members. Instead frame into floor diaphragms.

Windows

✔ Use the thinnest glass section that is acceptable for conventional loads.

✔ Design window systems so that the frame anchorage and the supporting wall are capable of resisting the breaking pressure of the window glass.

✔ Use laminated annealed glass (for insulated panels, only the interior pane needs to be laminated).

✔ Design window frames with a minimum of a ½-inch bite.

✔ Use a minimum of a ¼-inch silicone sealant around the inside glass perimeter, with a minimum tensile strength of 20 psi.

6.4.5   Further Reading

Norville, H.S., Harville, N., Conrath, E.J., Shariat, S., and Mallone, S., 1999, Glass-Related Injuries in Oklahoma City Bombing, *Journal of Performance of Constructed Facilities*,Vol. 13, No. 2. http://www.pubs.asce.org/WWWdisplay.cgi?9902006

Emek, M. and Tennant, D., 1998, "Energy Absorbing Blast Mitigating Window Systems", *Glass Magazine*, McLean, Virginia.

Smilowitz, R. and Tennant, D., 1998, "Curtainwall Systems and Blast Loading," *Glass Magazine*, McLean, Virginia.

6.5   MECHANICAL AND ELECTRICAL SYSTEMS

In the event of an explosion directed at a high-occupancy building, the primary objective is to protect people by preventing building collapse. Secondary goals are to limit injuries due to flying building debris and the direct effects of air blast entering the building (i.e., impact due to being thrown or lung collapse). Beyond these life-safety concerns, the objective is to facilitate building evacuation and rescue efforts through effective building design. This last objective is the focus of this section. Issues related specifically to chemical, biological, and radiological threats are discussed under a separate section with that heading.

The key concepts for providing secure and effective mechanical and electrical systems in buildings is the same as for the other building systems: separation, hardening, and redundancy. Keeping critical mechanical and electrical functions as far from high-threat areas as possible (e.g., lobbies, loading docks, mail rooms, garages, and retail spaces) increases their ability to survive an event. Separation is perhaps the most cost-effective option. Additionally, physical hardening or protection of these systems (including the conduits, pipes, and ducts associated with life-safety systems) provides increased likelihood that they will be able to survive the direct effects of the event if they are close enough to be affected. Finally, by providing redundant emergency systems that are adequately separated, there is a greater likelihood that emergency systems will remain operational post-event to assist rescuers in the evacuation of the building.

Architecturally, enhancements to mechanical and electrical systems will require additional space to accommodate additional equipment. Fortunately, there are many incremental improvements that can be made that require only a small change to the design. Additional space can be provided for future enhancements as funds or the risk justify implementation.

Structurally, the walls and floor systems adjacent to the areas where critical equipment are located need to be protected by means of hardening. Other areas where hardening is recommended include primary egress routes, feeders for emergency power distribution, sprinkler systems mains and risers, fire alarm system trunk wiring, and ducts used for smoke-control systems.

From an operational security standpoint, it is important to restrict and control access to air-intake louvers, mechanical and electrical rooms, telecommunications spaces and rooftops by means of such measures as visitor screening, limited elevator stops, closed-circuit television (CCTV), detection, and card access-control systems.

Specific recommendations are given below for (1) emergency egress routes, (2) the emergency power system, (3) fuel storage, (4) transformers, (5) ventilation systems, (6) the fire control center, (7) emergency elevators, (8) the smoke and fire detection and alarm system, (9) the sprinkler/standpipe system, (10) smoke control system, and (11) the communication system. Air intakes are covered in Section 6.6.

6.5.1   Emergency Egress Routes

To facilitate evacuation consider these measures.

- Provide positive pressurization of stairwells and vestibules.
- Provide battery packs for lighting fixtures and exit signs.
- Harden walls using reinforced CMU block properly anchored at supports.

○ Use non-slip phosphorescent treads.

○ Do not cluster egress routes in single shaft. Separate them as far as possible.

○ Use double doors for mass evacuation.

○ Do not use glass along primary egress routes or stairwells.

6.5.2   Emergency Power System

An emergency generator provides an alternate source of power should utility power become unavailable to critical life-safety systems such as alarm systems, egress lighting fixtures, exit signs, emergency communications systems, smoke-control equipment, and fire pumps.

Emergency generators typically require large louvers to allow for ventilation of the generator while running. Care should be taken to locate the generator so that these louvers are not vulnerable to attack. A remote radiator system could be used to reduce the louver size.

Redundant emergency generator systems remotely located from each other enable the supply of emergency power from either of two locations. Consider locating emergency power-distribution feeders in hardened enclosures, or encased in concrete, and configured in redundant routing paths to enhance reliability. Emergency distribution panels and automatic transfer switches should be located in rooms separate from the normal power system (hardened rooms, where possible).

Emergency lighting fixtures and exit signs along the egress path could be provided with integral battery packs, which locates the power source directly at the load, to provide lighting instantly in the event of a utility power outage.

6.5.3   Fuel storage

A non-explosive fuel source, such as diesel fuel, is acceptable for standby use for emergency generators and diesel fire pumps. Fuel tanks should be located away from building access points, in fire-rated, hardened enclosures. Fuel piping within the building should be located in hardened enclosures, and redundant piping systems could be provided to enhance the reliability of the fuel distribution system. Fuel filling stations should be located away from public access points and monitored by the CCTV system.

6.5.4   Transformers

Main power transformer(s) should be located interior to the building if possible, away from locations accessible to the public. For larger buildings, multiple transformers, located remotely from each other, could enhance reliability should one transformer be damaged by an explosion.

6.5.5   Ventilation Systems

Air-intake locations should be located as high up in the building as is practical to limit access to the general public. Systems that serve public access areas such as mail receiving rooms, loading docks, lobbies, freight elevators/lobbies should be isolated and provided with dedicated air handling systems capable of 100 percent exhaust mode. Tie air intake locations and fan rooms into the security surveillance and alarm system.

Building HVAC systems are typically controlled by a building automation system, which allows for quick response to shut down or selectively control air conditioning systems. This system is coordinated with the smoke-control and fire-alarm systems.

See Section 6.6 on chemical, biological, and radiological protection for more information.

6.5.6   Fire Control Center

A Fire Control Center should be provided to monitor alarms and life-safety components, operate smoke-control systems, communicate with occupants, and control the fire-fighting/evacuation process. Consider providing redundant Fire Control Centers remotely located from each other to allow system operation and control from alternate locations. The Fire Control Center should be located near the point of firefighter access to the building. If the control center is adjacent to lobby, separate it from the lobby using a corridor or other buffer area. Provide hardened construction for the Fire Control Center.

6.5.7   Emergency Elevators

Elevators are not used as a means of egress from a building in the event of a life-safety emergency event, as conventional elevators are not suitably protected from the penetration of smoke into the elevator shaft. An unwitting passenger could be endangered if an elevator door opens onto a smoke filled lobby. Firefighters may elect to manually use an elevator for firefighting or rescue operation.

A dedicated elevator, within its own hardened, smoke-proof enclosure, could enhance the firefighting and rescue operation after a blast/fire event. The dedicated elevator should be supplied from the emergency generator, fed by conduit/wire that is protected in hardened enclosures. This shaft/lobby assembly should be sealed and positively pressurized to prevent the penetration of smoke into the protected area.

6.5.8 Smoke and Fire Detection and Alarm System

A combination of early-warning smoke detectors, sprinkler-flow switches, manual pull stations, and audible and visual alarms provide quick response and notification of an event. The activation of any device will automatically start the sequence of operation of smoke control, egress, and communication systems to allow occupants to quickly go to a safe area. System designs should include redundancy such as looped infrastructure wiring and distributed intelligence such that the severing of the loop will not disable the system.

Install a fire-alarm system consisting of distributed intelligent fire alarm panels connected in a peer-to-peer network, such that each panel can function independently and process alarms and initiate sequences within its respective zone.

6.5.9 Sprinkler/Standpipe System

Sprinklers will automatically suppress fire in the area upon sensing heat. Sprinkler activation will activate the fire alarm system. Standpipes have water available locally in large quantities for use by professional fire fighters. Multiple sprinkler and standpipe risers limit the possibility of an event severing all water supply available to fight a fire.

Redundant water services would increase the reliability of the source for sprinkler protection and fire suppression. Appropriate valving should be provided where services are combined.

Redundant fire pumps could be provided in remote locations. These pumps could rely on different sources, for example one electric pump supplied from the utility and/or emergency generator and a second diesel fuel source fire pump.

Diverse and separate routing of standpipe and sprinkler risers within hardened areas will enhance the system's reliability (i.e., reinforced masonry walls at stair shafts containing standpipes).

6.5.10 Smoke-Control Systems

Appropriate smoke-control systems maintain smoke-free paths of egress for building occupants through a series of fans, ductwork, and fire-smoke dampers. Stair pressurization systems maintain a clear path of egress for occupants to safe areas or to evacuate the building. Smoke-control fans should be located higher in a building rather than at lower floors to limit exposure/access to external vents. Vestibules at stairways with separate pressurization provide an additional layer of smoke control.

6.5.11 Communication System

A voice communication system facilitates the orderly control of occupants and evacuation of the danger area or the entire building. The system is typically zoned by floor, by stairwell, and by elevator bank for selective communication to building occupants.

Emergency communication can be enhanced by providing

- extra emergency phones separate from the telephone system, connected directly to a constantly supervised central station;
- in-building repeater system for police, fire, and EMS (Emergency Medical Services) radios; and
- redundant or wireless fireman's communications in building.

6.5.12 Checklist – Mechanical and Electrical Systems

✔ Place all emergency functions away from high-risk areas in protected locations with restricted access.

✔ Provide redundant and separated emergency functions.

✔ Harden and/or provide physical buffer zones for the enclosures around emergency equipment, controls, and wiring.

✔ For egress routes, provide battery packs for exit signs, use non-slip phosphorescent treads, and double doors for mass evacuation.

✔ Avoid using glass along primary egress routes or stairwells.

✔ Place emergency functions away from structurally vulnerable areas such as transfer girders.

✔ Place a transformer interior to building, if possible.

✔ Provide access to the fire control center from the building exterior.

6.5.13   Further Reading

Building Owners and Managers Association International, 1996, *How to Design and Manage Your Preventive Maintenance Program*, Building Owners and Managers Association International, Washington, D.C. http://www.boma.org/pubs/bomapmp.htm

Kurtz,N.D., Hlushko, A., and Nall, D., 2002, Engineering Systems and an Incremental Response to Terrorist Threat, *Building Standards Magazine*, July-August 2002, Whittier, California, pages 24-27.

Craighead, G., 2002, *High-Rise Security and Fire Life Safety, 2nd Edition*, Academic Press, ISBN 0750674555 http://www.amazon.com/exec/obidos/tg/detail/-/0750674555/qid=/br=1-/ref=br_lf_b_//t/103-7416668-4182264?v=glance&s=books&n=173507#product-details

Council on Tall Buildings and Urban Habitat, 2001, *Task Force on Tall Buildings: "The Future,"* Council on Tall Buildings and Urban Habitat, Lehigh University, Bethlehem, Pennsylvania. http://www.lehigh.edu/ctbuh/htmlfiles/hot_links/report.pdf

6.6   CHEMICAL, BIOLOGICAL, AND RADIOLOGICAL PROTECTION

This section discusses three types of air-borne hazards.

1. A large exterior release originating some distance away from the building (includes delivery by aircraft).

2. A small localized exterior release at an air intake or other opening in the exterior envelope of the building.

3. A small interior release in a publicly accessible area, a major egress route, or other vulnerable area (e.g., lobby, mail room, delivery receiving).

Like explosive threats, chemical, biological and radiological (CBR) threats may be delivered externally or internally to the building. External ground-based threats may be released at a standoff distance from the building or may be delivered directly through an air intake or other opening. Interior threats may be delivered to accessible areas such as the lobby, mailroom, or loading dock, or they may be released into a secured area such as a primary egress route. This discussion is limited to air-borne hazards.

There may not be an official or obvious warning prior to a CBR event. While you should always follow any official warnings, the best defense is to be alert to signs of a release occurring near you. The air may be contaminated if you see a suspicious cloud or smoke near ground level, hear an air blast, smell strange odors, see birds or other small animals dying, or hear of more than one person complaining of eye, throat or skin irritation or convulsing.

Chemicals will typically cause problems within in seconds or minutes after exposure, but they can sometimes have delayed effects that will not appear for hours or days. Symptoms may include blurred or dimmed vision; eye, throat, or skin irritation; difficulty breathing; excess saliva; or nausea.

Biological and some radioactive contaminants typically will take days to weeks before symptoms appear, so listen for official information regarding symptoms.

With radioactive "dirty" bombs, the initial risk is from the explosion. Local responders may advise you to either shelter-in-place or evacuate. After the initial debris falls to the ground, leaving the area and washing will minimize your risk from the radiation.

Buildings provide a limited level of inherent protection against CBR threats. To some extent, the protection level is a function of how airtight the building is, but to a greater extent it is a function of the HVAC system's design and operating parameters.

The objectives of protective building design as they relate to the CBR threat are first to make it difficult for the terrorist to successfully execute a CBR attack and second, to minimize the impact (e.g., life, health, property damage, loss of commerce) of an attack if it does occur.

In order to reduce the likelihood of an attack, use security and design features that limit the terrorist's ability to approach the building and successfully release the CBR contaminant. Some examples are listed below.

- Use security stand-off, accessibility, and screening procedures similar to those identified in the explosive threat mitigation sections of this document (see Chapter 5, Design Approach and Section 6.1, Site Location and Layout).

- Recognize areas around HVAC equipment and other mechanical systems to be vulnerable areas requiring special security considerations.

- Locate outdoor air intakes high above ground level and at inaccessible locations.

- Prevent unauthorized access to all mechanical areas and equipment.

- Avoid the use of ground-level mechanical rooms accessible from outside the building. Where such room placement is unavoidable, doors and air vents leading to these rooms should be treated as vulnerable locations and appropriately secured.

- Treat operable, ground-level windows as a vulnerability and either avoid their use or provide appropriate security precautions to minimize the vulnerability.

- Interior to the building, minimize public access to HVAC return-air systems.

Further discussion of some of these prevention methods is provided below.

6.6.1   Air intakes

Air intakes may be made less accessible by placing them as high as possible on the building exterior, with louvers flush with the exterior (see figure 6-9). All opportunities to reach air-intakes through climbing should be eliminated. Ideally, there is a vertical smooth surface from the ground level to the intake louvers, without such features as high shrubbery, low roofs, canopies, or sunshades, as these features can enable climbing and concealment. To prevent opportunities for a weapon to be lobbed into the intake, the intake louver should be ideally flush with the wall. Otherwise, a surface sloped at least 45 degrees away from the building and further protected through the use of metal mesh (a.k.a. bird screen) should be used. Finally, CCTV surveillance and enhanced security is recommended at intakes.

In addition to providing protection against an air-borne hazard delivered directly into the building, placing air-intakes high above ground provides protection against ground-based standoff threats because the concentration of the air-borne hazard diminishes somewhat with height. Because air-blast pressure decays with height, elevated air intakes also provide modest protection against explosion threats. Furthermore, many recognized sources of indoor air contaminants (e.g., vehicle exhaust, standing water, lawn chemicals, trash, and rodents) tend to be located near ground level. Thus, elevated air intakes are a recommended practice in general for providing healthy indoor air quality.

In the event that a particular air intake does not service an occupied area, it may not be necessary to elevate it above ground level. However,

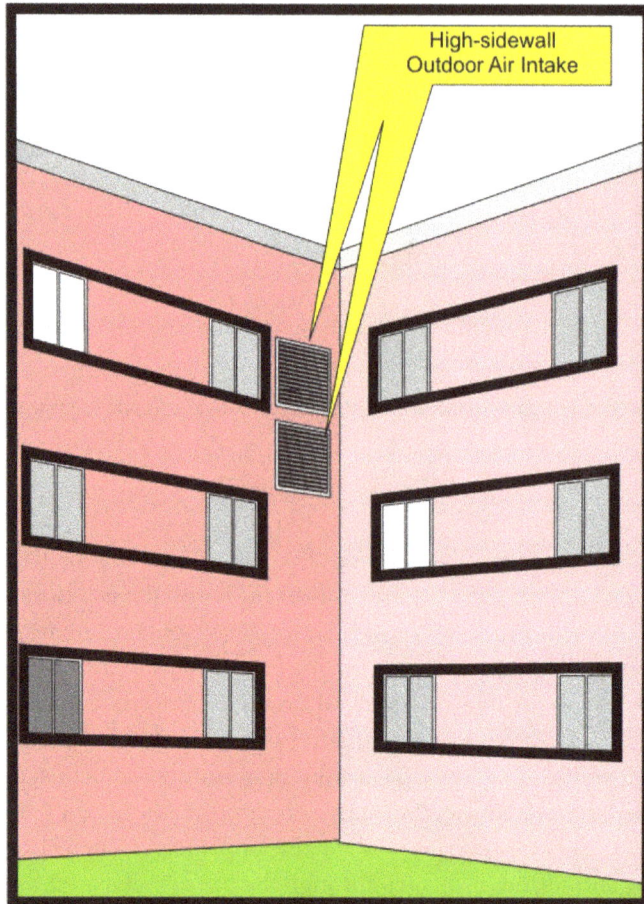

High-sidewall
Outdoor Air Intake

Figure 6-9   Schematic showing recommended location for elevated air-
               intakes on exterior of building.

if the unoccupied area is within an otherwise occupied building, the
intake should either be elevated or significant precautions (tightly
sealed construction between unoccupied/occupied areas, unoccupied
area maintained at negative pressure relative to occupied area) should
be put in place to ensure that contaminants are unable to penetrate
into the occupied area of the building.

6.6.2 Mechanical Areas

Another simple measure is to tightly restrict access to building mechanical areas (e.g., mechanical rooms, roofs, elevator equipment access).
These areas provide access to equipment and systems (e.g., HVAC, elevator, building exhaust, and communication and control) that could be

used or manipulated to assist in a CBR attack. Additional protection may be provided by including these areas in those monitored by electronic security and by eliminating elevator stops at the levels that house this equipment. For rooftop mechanical equipment, ways of restricting (or at least monitoring) access to the roof that do not violate fire codes should be pursued.

6.6.3   Return-Air Systems

Similar to the outdoor-air intake, HVAC return-air systems inside the building can be vulnerable to CBR attack. Buildings requiring public access have an increased vulnerability to such an attack. Design approaches that reduce this vulnerability include the use of ducted HVAC returns within public access areas and the careful placement of return-air louvers in secure locations not easily accessed by public occupants.

The second objective is to design to minimize the impact of an attack. For many buildings, especially those requiring public access, the ability to prevent a determined terrorist from initiating a CBR release will be a significant challenge. Compared to buildings in which campus security and internal access can be strictly controlled, public-access buildings may require a greater emphasis on mitigation. However, even private-access facilities can fall victim to an internal CBR release, whether through a security lapse or perhaps a delivered product (mail, package, equipment, or food). Examples of design methods to minimize the impact of a CBR attack are listed below.

- Public access routes to the building should be designed to channel pedestrians through points of noticeable security presence.
- The structural and HVAC design should isolate the most vulnerable public areas (entrance lobbies, mail rooms, load/delivery docks) both physically and in terms of potential contaminant migration.
- The HVAC and auxiliary air systems should carefully use positive and negative pressure relationships to influence contaminant migration routes.

Further discussion of some of these prevention methods is provided below.

6.6.4   Lobbies, Loading Docks, and Mail Sorting Areas

Vulnerable internal areas where airborne hazards may be brought into the building should be strategically located. These include lobbies, loading docks, and mail sorting areas. Where possible, place these functions outside of the footprint of the main building. When incorporated into the main building, these areas should be physically separated from other areas by floor-to-roof walls. Additionally, these areas should be maintained under negative pressure relative to the rest of the building, but at positive-to-neutral pressure relative to the outdoors. To assist in maintaining the desired pressure relationship, necessary openings (doors, windows, etc.) between secure and vulnerable areas should be equipped with sealing windows and doors, and wall openings due to ductwork, utilities, and other penetrations should be sealed. Where entries into vulnerable areas are frequent, the use of airlocks or vestibules may be necessary to maintain the desired pressure differentials.

Ductwork that travels through vulnerable areas should be sealed. Ideally, these areas should have separate air-handling units to isolate the hazard. Alternatively, the conditioned air supply to these areas may come from a central unit as long as exhaust/return air from these areas is not allowed to mix into other portions of the building. In addition, emergency exhaust fans that can be activated upon internal CBR release within the vulnerable area will help to purge the hazard from the building and minimize its migration into other areas. Care must be taken that the discharge point for the exhaust system is not co-located with expected egress routes. Consideration should also be given to filtering this exhaust with High Efficiency Particulate Air (HEPA) filtration. For entrance lobbies that contain a security screening location, it is recommended that an airlock or vestibule be provided between the secured and unsecured areas.

6.6.5   Zoning of HVAC Systems

Large buildings usually have multiple HVAC (heating, ventilation, air-conditioning) zones, each zone with its own air-handling unit and duct system. In practice, these zones are not completely separated if they are on the same floor. Air circulates among zones through plenum returns, hallways, atria, and doorways that are normally left open. Depending upon the HVAC design and operation, airflow between zones on different floors can also occur through the intentional use of shared air-return/supply systems and through air migrations via stairs and elevator shafts.

Isolating the separate HVAC zones minimizes the potential spread of an airborne hazard within a building, reducing the number of people potentially exposed if there is an internal release. Zone separation also provides limited benefit against an external release, as it increases internal resistance to air movement produced by wind forces and chimney effect, thus reducing the rate of infiltration. In essence, isolating zones divides the building into separate environments, limiting the effects of a single release to an isolated portion of the building. Isolation of zones requires full-height walls between each zone and the adjacent zones and hallway doors.

Another recommendation is to isolate the return system (i.e., no shared returns). Strategically locate return air grills in easily observable locations and preferably in areas with reduced public access.

Both centralized and decentralized shutdown capabilities are advantageous. To quickly shut down all HVAC systems at once in the event of an external threat, a single-switch control is recommended for all air-exchange fans (includes bathroom, kitchen, and other exhaust sources). In the event of a localized internal release, redundant decentralized shutdown capability is also recommended. Controls should be placed in a location easily accessed by the facility manager, security, or emergency response personnel. Duplicative and separated control systems will add an increased degree of protection. Further protection may be achieved by placing low-leakage automatic dampers on air intakes and exhaust fans that do not already have back-draft dampers.

6.6.6   Positive Pressurization

Traditional good engineering practice for HVAC design strives to achieve a slight overpressure of 5-12 Pa (.02-inch-.05-inch w.g.) within the building environment, relative to the outdoors. This design practice is intended to reduce uncontrolled infiltration into the building. When combined with effective filtration, this practice will also provide enhanced protection against external releases of CBR aerosols.

Using off-the-shelf technology (e.g., HEPA), manually triggered augmentation systems can be put into place to over-pressure critical zones to intentionally impact routes of contaminant migration and/or to provide safe havens for sheltering-in-place. For egress routes, positive-pressurization is also recommended, unless of course, the CBR source is placed within the egress route. Design parameters for such systems will depend upon many factors specific to the building and critical zone in question. Care must be taken that efforts to obtain a desired pressure relationship within one zone, will not put occupants in another zone at increased risk. Lastly, the supply air used to pressurize the critical space must be appropriately filtered (see filtration discussion below) or originate from a non-contaminated source in order to be beneficial.

6.6.7   Airtightness

To limit the infiltration of contaminants from outside the building into the building envelope, building construction should be made as airtight as possible. Tight construction practices (weatherization techniques, tightly sealing windows, doors, wall construction, continuous vapor barriers, sealing interface between wall and window/door frames) will also help to maintain the desired pressure relationships between HVAC zones. To ensure that the construction of the building has been performed correctly, building commissioning is recommended throughout the construction process and prior to taking ownership to observe construction practices and to identify potential airflow trouble spots (cracks, seams, joints, and pores in the building envelope and along the lines separating unsecured from secured space) before they are covered with finish materials.

6.6.8   Filtration Systems

To offer effective protection, filtration systems should be specific to the particular contaminant's physical state and size. Chemical vapor/gas filtration (a.k.a. air cleaning) is currently a very expensive task (high initial and recurring costs) with a limited number of design professionals experienced in its implementation. Specific expertise should be sought if chemical filtration is desired. Possible application of the air cleaning approach to collective protection zones (with emergency activation) can assist in significantly reducing the cost though the protection is limited to the reduced size of the zone.

Most "traditional" HVAC filtration systems focus on aerosol type contaminants. The CBR threats in this category include radioactive "dirty bombs", bio-aerosols, and some chemical threats. Riot-control agents and low-volatility nerve agents, for example, are generally distributed in aerosol form; however, a vapor component of these chemical agents could pass through a filtration system. HEPA filtration is currently considered adequate by most professionals to achieve sufficient protection from CBR particulates and aerosols. However, HEPA filtration systems generally have a higher acquisition cost than traditional HVAC filters and they cause larger pressure drops within the HVAC system, resulting in increased energy requirements to maintain the same design airflow rate. Due to recent improvements in filter media development, significant improvements in aerosol filtration can be achieved at relatively minimal increases in initial and operating costs. Also important is that incremental increases in filtration efficiency will generally provide incremental increases in protection from the aerosol contaminant.

In 1999, the American Society of Heating, Refrigeration, and Air Conditioning Engineers (ASHRAE) released Standard 52.2-1999. This standard provides a system for rating filters that quantifies filtration efficiency in different particle size ranges to provide a composite efficiency value named the Minimum Efficiency Reporting Value (MERV). MERV ratings range between 1 and 20 with a higher MERV indicating a more efficient filter. Using the MERV rating table, a desired filter efficiency may be selected according to the size of the contaminant under consideration. For example, a filter with a MERV of 13 or more will provide a 90% or greater reduction of most CBR aerosols (generally considered to be at least 1-3 um in size or larger) within the filtered airstream with much lower acquisition and maintenance costs than HEPA filtration.

Efficiency of filtration systems is not the only concern. Air can become filtered only if it actually passes through the filter. Thus, filter-rack design, gasketing, and good quality filter sources should all play a role in minimizing bypass around the filter. The use of return-air filtration systems and the strategic location of supply and return systems should also be carefully employed to maximize effective ventilation and filtration rates.

6.6.9 Detection Systems

Beyond the measures discussed above, there is the option of using detection systems as part of the protective design package. In general, affordable, timely, and practical detection systems specific to all CBR agents are not yet available. However, for aerosol contaminants, non-specific detection equipment can be employed to activate response actions should a sudden spike in aerosol concentration of a specific size range be detected. If the spike were detected in an outdoor intake for example, this could trigger possible response options such as damper closure, system shutdown, bypass to alternate air intake, or rerouting the air through a special bank of filters. Such protective actions could occur until an investigation was performed by trained personnel (i.e., check with adjacent alarms, and review security tape covering outdoor air intake). Unless foul play was discovered, the entire process could be completed within 10 minutes or less and without alarming occupants. The initial cost of such a system is relatively modest (depending upon the number of detectors and response options incorporated into the design), but the maintenance requirements are relatively high. Similar monitoring systems could be employed to trigger appropriate responses in high-threat areas such as mailrooms, shipping/receiving areas, or entrance lobbies. The approach could also be expanded to incorporate some of the newer chemical detection technologies, though the low threshold requirements may generate a substantial number of false positives. As technology progresses, detector availability and specificity should continue to expand into the general marketplace.

It is recognized that at this time, detection systems are not appropriate for many buildings. Consider using higher-efficiency filtration systems initially and design HVAC systems so that detection systems can be easily integrated into the HVAC control package at a later date.

6.6.10 Emergency Response Using Fire/HVAC Control Center

Certain operations that are managed at the Fire Control Center can play a protective role in the response to a CBR incident. Examples of such operations and how they could be used are given below.

○ **Purge fans.** These can be used to purge an interior CBR release or to reduce indoor contaminant concentrations following building exposure to an external CBR source. (Note: In practice, some jurisdictions may recommend purging for chemical and radiological contaminants but not for biological contaminants, which may be communicable and/or medically treatable.)

○ **Communication Systems.** Building communication systems that allow specific instructions to be addressed to occupants in specific zones of the building can play a significant role in directing occupant response to either an internal or external release.

○ **Pressurization Fans.** These provide two functions. First, the ability to override and deactivate specific positive-pressure zones may be beneficial in the event that a known CBR source is placed into such an area. Second, areas designated for positive pressurization (generally for smoke protection) may also become beneficial havens for protection from internal and external CBR releases, if they are supplied by appropriately filtered air.

○ **HVAC Controls.** The ability to simultaneous and individually manipulate operation of all HVAC and exhaust equipment from a single location may be very useful during a CBR event. Individuals empowered to operate such controls must be trained in their use.

The provision of simple floor-by-floor schematics showing equipment locations and the locations of supply and return louvers will aid the utility of this control option.

○ **Elevator Controls.** Depending upon their design and operation, the ability to recall elevators to the ground floor may assist in reducing contaminant migration during a CBR event.

6.6.11   Evolving Technologies

Many of the challenges relating to CBR terrorism prevention will be facilitated with the introduction of new technologies developed to address this emerging threat. As vendors and products come to market, it is important that the designer evaluate performance claims with a close level of scrutiny. Vendors should be willing to guarantee performance specs in writing, provide proof of testing (and show certified results) by an independent, reputable lab, and the testing conditions (e.g., flow rate, residence time, incoming concentrations) should be consistent with what would be experienced within the owner's building. For CBR developments, proof of federal government testing and acceptance may be available.

6.6.12   Checklist – Chemical, Biological & Radiological Protective Measures

✔ Place air intakes servicing occupied areas as high as practically possible (minimum 12 feet above ground). GSA may require locating at fourth floor or above when applicable.

✔ Restrict access to critical equipment.

✔ Isolate separate HVAC zones and return air systems.

✔ Isolate HVAC supply and return systems in unsecured areas.

✔ Physically isolate unsecured areas from secured areas.

✔ Use positive pressurization of primary egress routes, safe havens, and/or other critical areas.

✔ Commission building throughout construction and prior to taking ownership.

✔ Provide redundant, easily accessible shutdown capabilities.

✔ For higher levels of protection, consider using contaminant-specific filtration and detection systems.

✔ Incorporate fast-acting, low-leaking dampers.

✔ Filter both return air and outdoor air for publicly accessible buildings.

✔ Select filter efficiencies based upon contaminant size. Use reputable filter media installed into tight-fitting, gasketed, and secure filter racks.

✔ For higher threat areas (mail room, receiving, reception/screening lobby):

  ○ Preferably locate these areas outside the main building footprint.

  ○ Provide separate HVAC, with isolated returns capable of 100% exhaust.

  ○ Operate these areas at negative pressure relative to secure portion of the building.

  ○ Use air-tight construction, vestibules, and air locks if there is high traffic flow.

  ○ Consider installation of an emergency exhaust fan to be activated upon suspected internal CBR release.

✔ Lock, secure, access-log, and control mechanical rooms.

✔ In public access areas, use air diffusers and return air grills that are secure or under security observation.

✔ Zone the building communication system so that it is capable of delivering explicit instructions, and has back-up power.

✔ Create safe zones using enhanced filtration, tight construction, emergency power, dedicated communication systems, and appropriate supplies (food, water, first aide, and personal-protective equipment).

6.6.13 Further Reading

Miller, J., 2002, Defensive Filtration, *ASHRAE Journal*, Vol. 44, No. 12, pp. 18-23, December 2002.

American Society of Heating, Refrigerating, and Air Conditioning Engineers, 2002, *Risk Management Guidance for Health and Safety under Extraordinary Incidents.* ASHRAE Winter Meeting Report, January 12, 2002. http://xp20.ashrae.org/ABOUT/ Task_Force_RPT_12Jan02.pdf

Centers for Disease Control and Prevention / National Institute for Occupational Safety and Health, 2002, *Guidance for Protecting Building Environments from Airborne Chemical, Biological, or Radiological Attacks.* Publication No. 2002-139, Cincinnati, Ohio. www.cdc.gov/ niosh/bldvent/2002-139.html

Central Intelligence Agency, 1998. *Chemical, Biological, Radiological Incident Handbook.* Central Intelligence Agency, Washington, D.C. http://www.cia.gov/cia/publications/cbr_handbook/cbrbook.htm

American Society of Heating, Refrigerating and Air-Conditioning Engineers, 2003, *Report of Presidential Ad Hoc Committee for Building Health and Safety under Extraordinary Incidents on Risk Management Guidance for Health, Safety and Environmental Security under Extraordinary Incidents,* Washington, D.C. http://xp20.ashrae.org/about/extraordinary.pdf

Centers for Disease Control and Prevention / National Institute for Occupational Safety and Health, 2003. *Guidance for Filtration and Air-Cleaning Systems to Protect Building Environments from Airborne Chemical, Biological, and Radiological Attacks, Publication No. 2003-136,* Cincinnati, Ohio. http://www.cdc.gov/niosh/docs/2003-136/2003-136.html

7.1 OVERVIEW

The previous chapters have focused on the protective design of office buildings because this occupancy is one that has been of most concern within the public and private sectors to date. The concepts discussed, however, are largely applicable to any type of civilian building serving large numbers of people on a daily basis. This chapter considers the unique challenges associated with three other high-occupancy building types: multi-family residential buildings, commercial retail buildings, and light-industrial buildings. Protection of schools and hospitals is addressed in other FEMA reports and is not explicitly addressed here.

The uniqueness of these other occupancy types from the perspective of protective design is a function of many factors, including hours of peak usage, dominant population, size of building, and construction type.

For dual-use facilities such as those that incorporate both retail and commercial office uses, two important recommendations for the HVAC are:

- to provide separate HVAC zones; and
- to strictly adhere to isolation principles (that is, to treat any public area as equivalent to an entrance lobby in a single-use building).

7.2 MULTI-FAMILY RESIDENTIAL OCCUPANCY

Multi-family residential buildings are unique because they tend to house more elderly, handicapped, and children than do office build-ings, which tend to have more able-bodied occupants within working age (18-65). Office buildings of course can have a certain percentage of less-able-bodied populations, depending on the tenancy (e.g., medical offices, social services, or child care centers), and such populations need to be accounted for in the design of these buildings as well. In any case, the occupancy will have a major effect on the evacuation and res-cue efforts.

For multi-family residential buildings, it becomes more imperative that primary egress routes, including hallways leading to stairwells, remain as clear of debris and smoke as possible during the evacuation period. This criterion demands a higher level of protection than has been dis-cussed for office buildings. Some recommendations for providing enhanced protection to facilitate evacuation and rescue of distressed populations are listed below.

- Place hallways in a protected location away from the building exterior.
- Do not use glass in the hallways used for primary egress.
- Egress routes should lead to exits that are as far as possible from high-risk areas such as the lobby, mail room, and delivery entrance.
- Create pressurized safe havens in elevator vestibules and stairwells using tightly constructed, air-tight enclosures placed in a protected core area of the building.
- Emergency exits should be easily accessible by emergency vehicles and should be spacious enough to accommodate rescue workers entering the building as well as injured persons exiting the building.
- The side(s) of the building with emergency exits should be free of any canopies, overhanging balconies, or other ornamentation that may fall and block the exits.
- Emergency power should provide sufficient lighting and or phosphorescence to lead persons safely out of the building.
- Avoid using false ceilings in hallways. These can become falling debris that interferes with evacuation.
- Attach light fixtures to the floor system above to avoid hazardous debris in the exit path and to provide emergency lighting.

Multi-family residential construction is more likely than office building construction to incorporate flat plate/slab or pre-fabricated components and therefore tends to be more structurally vulnerable. To improve performance, robust connection detailing becomes paramount to ensure that the connections are not weaker than the members to which they are attached. Also, balconies are more common in multi-family residential buildings. These present a debris hazard due to their inherent instability and connection weakness.

7.3 COMMERCIAL RETAIL SPACE OCCUPANCY

Commercial retail space such as malls, movie theatres, hotels, night clubs, casinos, and other spaces that house large public populations gathering for shopping or entertainment have their own unique features that increase their vulnerability compared with that of office buildings. Often, these spaces are low-rise buildings that have large interior spaces with high, laterally unsupported walls, long-span roofs, and interior columns spaced relatively far apart. They are generally constructed using lightweight construction and may be prefabricated. This type of construction has little if any redundancy, which increases the structural vulnerability significantly.

The primary goal for this type of construction is to prevent progressive collapse of the building in response to a large-scale attack. Where possible, floor-to-floor height and bay spacing should be reduced, and lateral bracing of the columns and roof joists should be provided. Connections should be designed to be at least as strong as the members. Secondary structural framing systems further enhance protection. To limit laceration injuries, lamination of glass is recommended. Consider structural partition walls or shelving units placed within the space that will stop the roof system from falling directly on the occupants in the event of collapse. If this approach is used, take care that the partitions have sufficient lateral support so that they do not topple over.

In these large spaces, it is virtually impossible to isolate HVAC to protect against CBR-type threats. In this case, negative zone pressurization or smoke-evacuation methods become critically important. Also, mechanical areas should be protected with restricted access and a hardened shell (walls, ceiling and floor). It is also recommended to have centralized redundant control stations, easily accessible by appropriate personnel. Consideration should be given to providing additional, clearly marked, easily located egress routes to facilitate mass evacuation. If there are business offices serving these buildings with a sizable workforce, consider relocating these and other mixed-use functions to a separate, offsite location.

7.4   LIGHT INDUSTRIAL BUILDINGS

Light industrial buildings are used through out the United States for offices, light manufacturing, laboratories, warehouses, and other commercial purposes. Typically, these buildings are low-rise buildings three to five stories high, often using tilt-up concrete construction. Typically, they are located in industrial or commercial complexes and may have significant setbacks from public streets. They are serviced by surface parking lots or parking structures outside the building. Security may vary widely depending on the use of the building. For a building used for laboratories or manufacturing, there may be already be significant security measures at the perimeter and inside the building. For office buildings, security may be light to negligible.

The main focus of this section is on light industrial buildings that house office space, because these are the buildings with potentially high populations, and therefore, life safety is a primary concern. For warehouses and manufacturing plants, the primary objective is more likely to be protection of the contents and processes. For laboratories, the primary objectives are to prevent release or deflagration of hazardous materials and to protect processes.

Office parks inherently have an open character with medium-to-large setbacks from the street and public parking. In this environment, the most effective way to protect the building from moving vehicle threats is to use landscaping methods between public streets and parking to prevent the intrusion of vehicles. Devices such as ponds, fountains, berms, and ditches can be very effective in reducing the accessibility of the building exterior to high-speed vehicles.

Parking should be placed as far as practical from the building. Driveways leading directly to the building entrance should have a meandering path from the public streets that does not permit high velocities to be achieved. Separation between the driveway and building may be achieved through a number of devices such as a pond with a bridge leading to the entrance, a knee wall with foliage in front, or other landscape features.

The design of parking structures servicing these buildings should fulfill two main objectives to prevent explosions in the parking structure from seriously damaging the main office building. The first is to control the lines of sight between the parking structure and the building to limit air-blast effects on the building. One solution is to use a solid wall that is bermed and landscaped on the side of the parking structure facing the building. Second, design the parking structure to withstand the design-level explosion without structural failure in order to reduce the potential for debris from a parking structure failure damaging the office building. This second objective can be achieved while still allowing the parking structure to sustain significant levels of damage.

For the tilt-up walls, use continuous vertical reinforcement with staggered splices, preferably on both sides of the wall to resist large lateral loads. It may be advantageous to consider designs that permit the wall to bear against floor diaphragms to resist loads. Connections between the walls and structural frame should be able to accept large rebound forces to prevent the wall from being pulled off the exterior. Care should be taken to prevent the wall from bearing directly against exterior columns to limit the opportunity for progressive collapse. Using laminated glass on the exterior reduces the potential for laceration injuries. For the roof, a concrete slab with or without decking is preferred over a solution using metal decking only.

7.5 FURTHER READING

FEMA, 1988, *Seismic Considerations: Office Buildings, FEMA 153, Earthquake Hazards Reduction Series 38,* Federal Emergency Management Agency, Washington, D.C.

FEMA, 1988, *Seismic Considerations: Apartment Buildings, FEMA 152, Earthquake Hazards Reduction Series 37.* Federal Emergency Management Agency, Washington, D.C.

8.1 INITIAL COSTS

The initial construction cost of protection has two components: fixed and variable. Fixed costs include such items as security hardware and space requirements. These costs do not depend on the level of an attack; that is, it costs the same to keep a truck away from a building whether the truck contains 500 or 5000 lbs. of TNT. Blast protection, on the other hand, is a variable cost. It depends on the threat level, which is a function of the explosive charge weight and the stand-off distance. Building designers have no control over the amount of explosives used, but are able to define a stand-off distance by providing a secured perimeter.

The optimal stand-off distance is determined by defining the total cost of protection as the sum of the cost of protection (construction cost) and the cost of stand-off (land cost). These two costs are considered as a function of the stand-off for a given explosive charge weight. The cost of protection is assumed to be proportional to the peak pressure at the building envelope, and the cost of land is a function of the square of the stand-off distance. The optimal stand-off is the one that minimizes the sum of these costs.

If additional land is not available to move the secured perimeter farther from the building, the required floor area of the building can be distributed among additional floors. As the number of floors is increased, the footprint decreases, providing an increased stand-off distance. Balancing the increasing cost of the structure (due to the added floors) and the corresponding decrease in protection cost (due to added stand-off), it is possible to find the optimal number of floors to minimize the cost of protection.

These methods for establishing an optimum stand-off distance are generally used for the maximum credible explosive charge. If the cost of protection for this charge weight is not within the budgetary constraints, then the design charge weight must be modified. A study can be conducted to determine the largest explosive yield and corresponding level of protection that can be incorporated into the building, given the available budget.

Though it is difficult to assign costs to various upgrade measures because they vary based on the site specific design, some generalizations

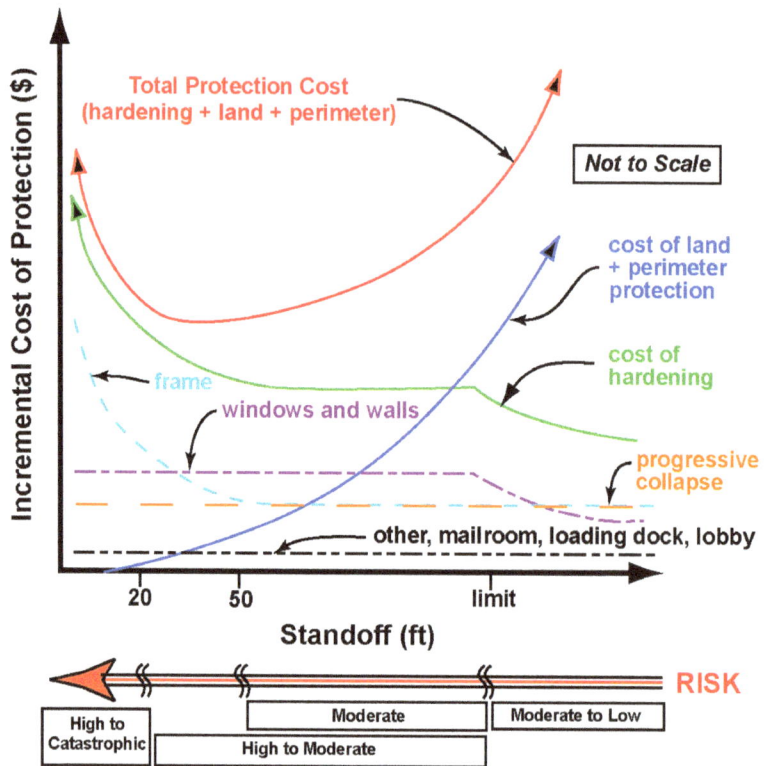

Figure 8-1   Plots showing relationship between cost of upgrading various building components, standoff distance, and risk

can be made (see Figure 8-1). Below is a list of enhancements arranged in order from least expensive to most expensive.

○ Hardening of unsecured areas

○ Measures to prevent progressive collapse

○ Exterior window and wall enhancements

8.2   LIFE-CYCLE COSTS

Life-cycle costs need to be considered as well. For example, if it is decided that two guarded entrances will be provided, one for the visitors and one for the employees, they may cost more during the life of the building than a single well designed entrance serving everyone. Also, maintenance costs may need to be considered. For instance the initial costs for a CBR detection system may be modest, but the maintenance costs are high. Finally, if the rentable square footage is reduced as a result of incorporating robustness into the building, this may have a large impact on the life-cycle costs.

8.3   SETTING PRIORITIES

If the costs associated with mitigating man-made hazards is too high, there are three approaches: (1) reduce the design threat, (2) increase the building setback, or (3) accept the risk. In some cases, the owner may decide to prioritize enhancements, based on their effectiveness in saving lives and reducing injuries. For instance, measures against progressive collapse are perhaps the most effective actions that can be implemented to save lives and should be considered above any other upgrades. Laminated glass is perhaps the single most effective measure to reduce extensive non-fatal injuries. If the cost is still considered too great, and the risk is high because of the location or the high-profile nature of the building, then the best option may be to consider building an unobtrusive facility in a lower-risk area instead. In some cases, for instance for financial institutions with trading floors, business interruption costs are so high they outweigh all other concerns. In such a case, the most cost-effective solution may be to provide a redundant facility.

Early consideration of man-made hazards will significantly reduce the overall cost of protection and increase the inherent protection level provided to the building. If protection measures are considered as an afterthought or not considered until the design is nearly complete, the cost is likely to be greater, because more areas will need to be structurally hardened due to poor planning. An awareness of the threat of man-made hazards from the beginning of a project also helps the team to decide early what the priorities are for the facility. For instance, if extensive teak paneling of interior areas visible from the exterior is desired by the architect for the architectural expression of the building, but the cost exceeds that of protective measures, than a decision needs to be made regarding the priorities of the project. Including protective measures as part of the discussion regarding trade-offs early in the design process often helps to clarify such issues.

Ultimately, the willingness to pay the additional cost for protection against man-made hazards is a function of the "probability of regrets" in the event a sizable incident occurs. In some situations, the small probability of an incident may not be compelling enough to institute these design enhancements. Using this type of logic, it is easy to see why it is unlikely that they will be instituted in any but the highest-risk buildings unless there is a mandated building code or insurance that requires these types of enhancements. This scenario is likely to lead to a selection process in which buildings stratify into two groups: those that incorporate no measures at all or only the most minimal provisions and those that incorporate high levels of protection. It also leads to the conclusion that it may not be appropriate to consider any but the most minimal measures for most buildings.

8.4 FURTHER READING

Bryant, L., & Smith, J., 2003, *Cost Impact of the ISC Security Criteria.* General Services Administration & Applied Research Associates, Inc., Vicksburg, Mississippi. http://www.oca.gsa.gov

Department of Defense, 1999, *Interim Antiterrorism/Force Protection Construction Standards.* [For Official Use Only]

Naval Facilities Engineering Service Center, 1998, *User's Guide on Security Glazing* Applications, UG-2030-SHR, Port Hueneme, California.

www.ingramcontent.com/pod-product-compliance
Lightning Source LLC
Chambersburg PA
CBHW081158270326
41930CB00014B/3201